Handbook of Atypical Parkinsonism

Handbook of Atypical Parkinsonism

Edited by

Carlo Colosimo
Consultant Neurologist and Professor,
Department of Neurology and Psychiatry,
Sapienza University of Rome, Italy

David E. Riley
Director, Movement Disorders Center, Department of Neurology,
Case Western Reserve University School of Medicine,
Cleveland, OH, USA

Gregor K. Wenning
Head, Division of Clinical Neurobiology, Movement Disorders Unit,
Department of Neurology, Medical University of Innsbruck, Austria

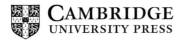

CAMBRIDGE
UNIVERSITY PRESS

CAMBRIDGE UNIVERSITY PRESS
Cambridge, New York, Melbourne, Madrid, Cape Town,
Singapore, São Paulo, Delhi, Tokyo, Mexico City

Cambridge University Press
The Edinburgh Building, Cambridge CB2 8RU, UK

Published in the United States of America by Cambridge University Press, New York

www.cambridge.org
Information on this title: www.cambridge.org/9780521111973

First published 2011

Printed in the United Kingdom at the University Press, Cambridge

A catalogue record for this publication is available from the British Library

Library of Congress Cataloguing in Publication data
Handbook of atypical parkinsonism / [edited by] Carlo Colosimo, David E. Riley,
    Gregor K. Wenning.
        p. ; cm.
    Includes bibliographical references and index.
    ISBN 978-0-521-11197-3 (hardback)
    1. Symptomatic Parkinson's disease.   I. Colosimo, Carlo.   II. Riley, David E.
    III. Wenning, Gregor K.   IV. Title.
    [DNLM: 1. Parkinsonian Disorders – diagnosis.   2. Diagnosis, Differential.
    3. Parkinsonian Disorders – therapy. WL 359]
    RC382.H34 2011
    616.8′33–dc22   2010042838

ISBN 978-0-521-11197-3 Hardback

Contents

Contributors

Marianna Amboni
Department of Neurological Sciences, University "Federico II," and IDC Hermitage-Capodimonte, Naples, Italy

Melissa J. Armstrong
Department of Medicine (Neurology), University of Toronto, ON, Canada

Paolo Barone
Department of Neurological Sciences, University "Federico II," Naples, Italy

Alfredo Berardelli
Department of Neurology and Psychiatry, Sapienza University of Rome, Italy

Bastiaan R. Bloem
Department of Neurology, Donders Centre for Brain, Cognition and Behaviour, Radboud University Nijmegen Medical Centre, The Netherlands

Carlo Colosimo
Department of Neurology and Psychiatry, Sapienza University of Rome, Italy

Giovanni Fabbrini
Department of Neurology and Psychiatry, Sapienza University of Rome, Italy

Roberta Granata
Division of Clinical Neurobiology, Department of Neurology, Medical University of Innsbruck, Austria

Johanna G. Kalf
Department of Rehabilitation, Division of Speech Language Pathology, Radboud University Nijmegen Medical Centre, The Netherlands

Anthony E. Lang
Department of Medicine (Neurology), University of Toronto, ON, Canada

Marten Munneke
Department of Neurology, Nijmegen Centre for Evidence Based Practice, Radboud University Nijmegen Medical Centre, The Netherlands

Maria Teresa Pellecchia
Department of Neurological Sciences, University "Federico II," Naples, Italy

David E. Riley
Movement Disorders Center, Department of Neurology, Case Western Reserve University School of Medicine, Cleveland, OH, USA

Gregor K. Wenning
Division of Clinical Neurobiology, Movement Disorders Unit, Department of Neurology, Medical University of Innsbruck, Austria

Preface

This defining handbook of atypical forms of parkinsonism continues a journey towards the understanding of pathogenesis, and ultimately the cure, of these rare, largely sporadic and universal diseases of late life.

It is a journey begun 50 years ago in Toronto by neurologist J Clifford Richardson, who recognized an unusual constellation of neurological symptoms in a friend. As Richardson puzzled about its features of progressive supranuclear palsy of gaze and bulbar muscles, axial dystonia, gait impairment and dementia, he identified 3 other patients with similar symptoms and realized their illness was an unrecognized neurodegenerative syndrome. He resisted opinions by neuropathologist colleagues that it was a variant of postencephalitic parkinsonism, and in 1962 he asked Jerzy Olszewski, the new professor of neuropathology at the Banting Institute, and me as his resident to examine the seven cases that were by then identified. We found the histopathology of neurofibrillary degeneration and gliosis in brainstem and subcortical nuclei was quite as distinctive as the clinical syndrome, but we could not be certain if it was a primary neurodegenerative disease like Alzheimer's, or an infection akin to scrapie which was just then beginning to be described.

Interest in progressive supranuclear palsy (PSP) has expanded since our description in 1964, and during the past 45 years its features have been vigorously investigated by an increasing number of neuroscientists using new biological techniques and studies that are facilitated by internet communication and international meetings. In 2010 we have learned PSP is a 4R tauopathy. Richardson's syndrome, as he originally described in 1963, is its principal manifestation but PSP disease also includes diverse phenotypes of isolated parkinsonism, corticobasal degeneration, pure akinesia, frontotemporal dementia and progressive nonfluent aphasia. Furthermore we have learned Richardson's syndrome is not unique to PSP disease, and it occurs also in (ALS)/Parkinsonism-dementia of Guam and in Guadeloupean parkinsonism.

As multiple system atrophy and corticobasal degeneration have been defined and studied in similar fashion to PSP, and as they are compared with the classical neurodegenerations of Parkinson's disease (PD), Alzheimer's disease (AD) and ALS, remarkable similarities are recognized between them.

All are featured by an abnormal and spreading protein that is specific to the neurodegeneration and accumulates in nerve cells and glia. Although some neurodegenerations are due to identified gene mutations, the majority are sporadic without obvious inheritance or family predisposition. Except for the 3 and 4R tauopathy of postencephalitic parkinsonism that followed encephalitis lethargica, and the spongiform encephalopathy of kuru that came after single feasts during mortuary cannibalism, there is no obvious preceding cause of these sporadic proteinopathies. Their onset is silent and asymptomatic, and it is not known if environmental exposure is single and isolated, or repeated and cumulative. It is not certain to what extent the pathogenesis could relate to genetic predisposition.

On Guam, a tropical island in the Western Pacific, the ALS/Parkinsonism-dementia complex (PDC) has held my interest for 27 years. It is a geographic isolate of a familial and long-latency polyproteinopathy that includes all the immunohistochemical proteins of all the major universal neurodegenerations. Its phenotypes are as diverse as its abnormal proteins, and include classical amyotrophic lateral sclerosis (ALS), PD, atypical parkinsonism with PSP and CBD, and Alzheimer-type dementia. During the past 50 years, this single disease has slowly declined by its principal phenotypes of ALS and PDC, and its age in onset has steadily increased. In 2010, classical ALS which was 100 times more common than elsewhere in 1953, no longer occurs on the island. Parkinsonism with dementia is uncommon and only 29 cases older than 70 were recently identified in a 2003 community survey of elderly Guamanians. The remarkable decline and disappearance of ALS/PDC in this distant place gives us hope that related and universal proteinopathies could end in the same way. But it is first necessary to identify its environmental cause and that remains our intention.

The challenge to Neurology in years ahead is to understand why abnormal proteins form, how they are acquired, and how each adversely affects the nervous system. We need to learn about their spread, and why the same protein can give rise to different phenotypes, and the same phenotype can be caused by different proteins. As we ask these questions, we will learn about protein metabolism and understand how we can influence and modify their abnormalities to prevent disease.

In 1964, we were not certain if PSP was a classical neurodegeneration akin to AD, or an infection due to a slow latent and temperate virus akin to scrapie. And we were aware of its similarities to postencephalitic parkinsonism. Forty-five years later we are still not certain. But we have learned that PSP and other neurodegenerations are due to the accumulation of abnormal proteins in the nervous system, and we are optimistic that future advances in understanding protein metabolism will give knowledge of pathogenesis and methods of cure.

I congratulate the editors for their fine presentation.

John Steele MD, FRCPC, FACP
Neurologist, Guam Memorial and US Navy Hospital

Introduction

Gregor K. Wenning, Carlo Colosimo, David E. Riley

Movement disorder experts are increasingly faced with atypical parkinsonism (AP) such as multiple system atrophy (MSA), progressive supranuclear palsy (PSP), or cortico-basal degeneration (CBD). Remarkably, these APs were all recognized during the 1960s. Historical milestones in the nosology and further understanding of these disorders are summarized in Table 1.1. Because of additional clinical features beyond the classic presentations of Parkinson's disease (PD), they have often been labeled "Parkinson-plus disorders." More recently, the term AP has come into vogue. The APs need to be distinguished from other causes of parkinsonism including PD, secondary forms of parkinsonism, and familial parkinsonism.

AP shares characteristics of parkinsonism, progressing more rapidly than PD and a poorly sustained or no response at all to levodopa, as well as additional atypical features (Table 1.2). As a consequence, the therapeutic approaches to these disorders differ substantially. MSA is characterized by early severe autonomic failure including orthostatic hypotension and urogenital failure. These symptoms are often neglected by neurologists, although they can be effectively treated in many patients. PSP patients with the classic clinical features (sometimes known as Richardson's syndrome) suffer from marked postural instability, requiring early provision of walking aids or wheelchairs to prevent the consequences of recurrent falls. In addition, such patients have severe vertical downgaze palsy. PSP patients with a more PD-like presentation show a more benign course with asymmetric parkinsonism, levodopa benefit, occasional levodopa-induced motor complications, with gaze and gait disturbances developing later. A third PSP phenotype is characterized by progressive speech, writing, and gait impairment with freezing unresponsive to levodopa therapy. CBD patients frequently exhibit asymmetric dystonic posturing of the hands and fingers, often associated with irregular myoclonic tremor. Other non-motor presentations of CBD such as progressive aphasia or cortical dementia are also commonly recognized.

Patients with PD may appear atypical when cognitive impairment is prominent. In these patients, parkinsonian features either precede (Parkinson's disease dementia, PDD) or follow (dementia with Lewy bodies, DLB) the dementia. PDD and DLB patients typically develop a progressive dementia syndrome characterized by fluctuating vigilance and psychosis, most often in the form of visual hallucinations. The psychotic symptoms may respond well to cholinesterase inhibitors. The levodopa response in DLB and particularly PDD is often comparable to that seen in PD. Autonomic failure may emerge in PD, PDD, and DLB; it should be treated like the dysautonomia of MSA.

Handbook of Atypical Parkinsonism, eds. Carlo Colosimo, David E. Riley, and Gregor K. Wenning.
Published by Cambridge University Press. © Cambridge University Press 2011.

Table 1.1   Historical milestones in atypical parkinsonism (reviewed by Stefanova et al. [17])

Multiple system atrophy

1900 Cerebellar presentation (Dejerine and Thomas [8])

1960 Autonomic presentation (Shy and Drager [9])

1961 Parkinson presentation (Adams *et al.* [10])

1969 Proposal of MSA as "umbrella" term (Graham and Oppenheimer [11])

1989 Glial cytoplasmic inclusions as cell marker of MSA (Papp *et al.* [12])

1989 First set of diagnostic criteria (Quinn [13])

1998 MSA is an α-synucleinopathy (Spillantini *et al.* [14])

1998 Consensus diagnostic criteria (Gilman *et al.* [15])

1999 Foundation of the European MSA Study Group (www.emsa-sg.org)

2004 Unified MSA Rating Scale (Wenning *et al.* [16])

2005 Transgenic MSA mouse models (Stefanova *et al.* [17])

2008 Revised Consensus diagnostic criteria (Gilman *et al.* [18])

2009 SNCA variants increase the risk for MSA (Scholz *et al.* [19])

2009 NNIPPS trial of riluzole in MSA (and PSP) patients (Bensimon *et al.* [20])

Dementia with Lewy bodies / Parkinson's disease dementia

1961 First report of DLB (Okazaki *et al.* [21])

1990 Lewy body variant of Alzheimer disease (Hansen *et al.* [22])

1993 Delineation of neuropathology in Lewy body disease (Kosaka [23])

1996 Diagnostic criteria for DLB (McKeith *et al.* [24])

1998 α-synuclein is a sensitive marker of DLB and PDD (Takeda *et al.* [25])

1998 Hereditary forms of DLB and PDD (Muenter *et al.* [26])

2000 Efficacy of rivastigmine in DLB (McKeith *et al.* [27])

2004 LRRK2 mutations in DLB (Zimprich *et al.* [28])

2004 Efficacy of rivastigmine in PDD (Emre *et al.* [29])

2005 Revision of diagnostic criteria for DLB (McKeith *et al.* [30])

2006 Glucocerebrosidase mutations in DLB (Goker-Alpan *et al.* [31])

2007 Diagnostic criteria for PDD (Emre *et al.* [32])

Progressive supranuclear palsy

1964 First report of PSP (Steele *et al.* [33])

1986 Filamentous tau is present in PSP brains (Pollock *et al.* [34])

1987 Pure akinesia (Imai *et al.* [35])

1987 First diagnostic criteria for PSP (Lees [36])

1996 NINDS-SPSP diagnostic criteria (Litvan *et al.* [37])

1998 PSP is a 4-repeat tauopathy (Mailliot *et al.* [38])

1999 PSP-like focus on Guadeloupe linked to tropical fruit (Caparros-Lefebvre *et al.* [39])

2001 PSP and CBD share a tau haplotype (Houlden *et al.* [40])

2005 Division of PSP into subtypes (Williams *et al.* [41])

2009 NNIPPS trial of riluzole in PSP (and MSA) patients (Bensimon *et al.* [20])

Table 1.1 (cont.)

Corticobasal degeneration
1968 First report of CBD (Rebeiz *et al.* [42])
1990 Premortem diagnosis of CBD (Riley *et al.* [43])
1994 Clinical diagnostic criteria (Lang *et al.* [44])
1999 Clinicopathological heterogeneity (Kertesz *et al.* [45])
2001 PSP and CBD share a tau haplotype (Houlden *et al.* [40])
2002 Neuropathological criteria (Dickson *et al.* [46])

Table 1.2 Selected features suggestive of atypical parkinsonism (modified from Quinn [47])

Motor
Rapid disease progression
Early instability and falls
Early freezing
Poor response to levodopa
Stimulus-sensitive myoclonus
Orofacial dystonia (spontaneous or levodopa-induced)
Camptocormia
Pisa syndrome
Disproportionate antecollis; retrocollis
Rocket sign
Procerus (corrugator supercilii) sign
Pyramidal signs
Cerebellar signs
Early dysarthria and dysphagia
Contractures
Severe fixed limb dystonia
Predominantly axial rigidity
Autonomic
Impotence / decreased genital sensitivity in females
Early and severe orthostatic hypotension
Absence of heart rate increase on standing
Early and severe urinary incontinence / incomplete bladder emptying
Fecal incontinence
Progressive anhidrosis
Nocturnal stridor
Cold hands sign
Extremity circulatory congestion
Oculomotor
Slowing of vertical saccades
Difficulty initiating saccades

Table 1.2 (cont.)

Supranuclear gaze palsy (particularly downgaze)

Gaze-evoked and positional downbeat nystagmus

Cognitive and neurobehavioral

Early and severe frontal dementia

Visual hallucinations not induced by medication

Ideomotor apraxia

Primary progressive aphasia

Cortical sensory loss

Sensory and/or visual neglect

Table 1.3 Classification of atypical parkinsonism according to protein aggregation

Synucleinopathies	Tauopathies
Parkinson's disease dementia	Progressive supranuclear palsy
Dementia with Lewy bodies	Richardson's syndrome
Multiple system atrophy	PSP-parkinsonism
Parkinsonian variant (MSA-P)	Pure akinesia
Cerebellar variant (MSA-C)	Corticobasal syndrome
	Frontotemporal lobar degeneration
	Apraxia of speech
	Corticobasal degeneration
	Corticobasal syndrome
	Frontotemporal dementia
	Progressive non-fluent aphasia

Until recently, the molecular pathology of AP remained elusive, preventing the development of effective therapeutic interventions. During the last ten years, fundamental insights into α-synuclein and tau genetics, and the pathology of AP have led to a new understanding of examples of this disorder as distinct proteinopathies (Table 1.3). Animal models based on transgenic expression of wild-type or mutated α-synuclein and tau genes have become available to further promote identification of pathogenic targets for drug development. Finally, newly developed and validated rating scales, natural history data, and improved MRI outcome measures provide the necessary framework for urgently needed intervention trials, several of which have been conducted already in DLB, MSA, and PSP patients. Therefore, it is increasingly important to discriminate PD from not only atypical parkinsonism generally but also from the various specific APs as early as possible. Figure 1.1 illustrates common features occurring in AP with diagnoses confirmed by postmortem examination.

The diagnosis of AP rests on criteria that have been validated for all disorders except for PDD and CBD. Diagnostic criteria for individual disorders are discussed in the various chapters. A definite diagnosis requires a postmortem examination showing typical cellular inclusions as well as selective neurodegeneration consistent with MSA, PDD DLB, PSP, or CBD. In 2003, a Scientific Issue Committee of the Movement Disorder Society analyzed the accuracy of the clinical diagnostic criteria available at that time [1]. Updated results are shown in Table 1.4. In retrospective validation studies, the criteria generally show good specificity, but poor sensitivity, particularly during early disease stages. Sensitivity increases during follow-up, but it remains suboptimal. In contrast, diagnostic accuracy can be improved

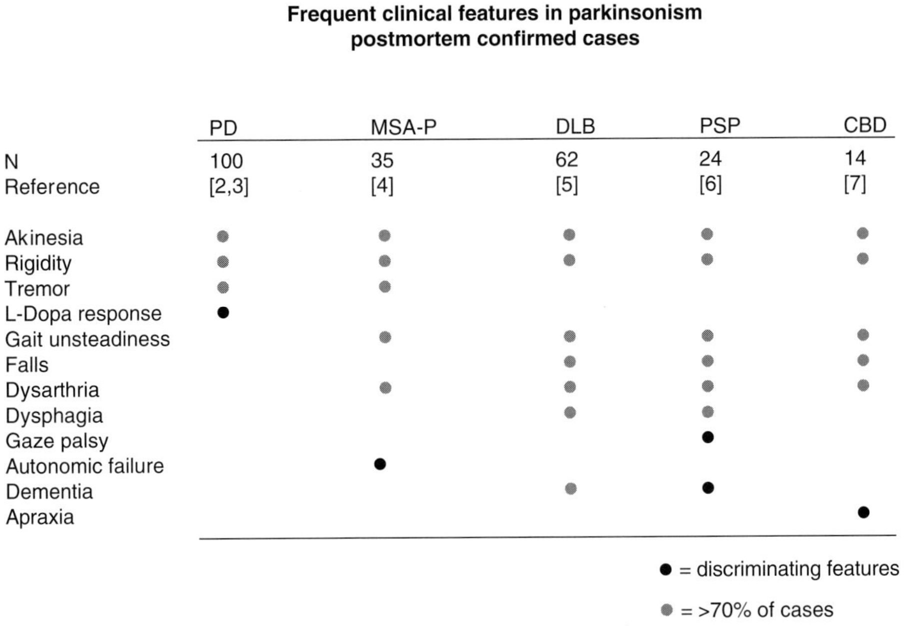

Frequent clinical features in parkinsonism postmortem confirmed cases

	PD	MSA-P	DLB	PSP	CBD
N	100	35	62	24	14
Reference	[2,3]	[4]	[5]	[6]	[7]
Akinesia	●	●	●	●	●
Rigidity	●	●	●	●	●
Tremor	●	●			
L-Dopa response	●				
Gait unsteadiness		●	●	●	●
Falls			●	●	●
Dysarthria		●	●	●	●
Dysphagia			●	●	
Gaze palsy				●	
Autonomic failure		●			
Dementia			●	●	
Apraxia					●

● = discriminating features

● = >70% of cases

Figure 1.1 Frequent clinical features occurring in atypical parkinsonism with diagnoses confirmed by postmortem examination.

Table 1.4 Validity of the clinical diagnostic criteria for progressive supranuclear palsy, multiple system atrophy, and dementia with Lewy bodies

(modified from Litvan et al. [1])

Disorder	Criteria	Sensitivity (%)	Specificity (%)	Positive predictive value (%)	Reference
PSP	NINDS possible 1st visit	83	93	83	36
	NINDS probable 1st visit	50	100	100	36
	NINDS possible 1st visit	21		100	48
	NINDS possible Last visit	85		83	48
	NINDS probable 1st visit	4		100	48

Table 1.4 (cont.)

Disorder	Criteria	Sensitivity (%)	Specificity (%)	Positive predictive value (%)	Reference
	NINDS probable Last visit	34		84	48
	QS MD Specialists Last visit	84	97	80	49
MSA	Revised Consensus Criteria possible 1st visit	41		95	50
	Revised Consensus Criteria possible Last visit	18		100	50
	Revised Consensus Criteria probable 1st visit	62		89	50
	Revised Consensus Criteria probable Last visit	63		91	50
	QS MD Specialists Last visit	88		86	49
DLB	McKeith 1st visit probable	18	99	75	51
	McKeith 2nd visit probable	29	99	56	51
	McKeith Possible*	83	91	92	30 a
	McKeith Probable*	83	95	96	30 a

* NINDS, National Institute of Neurological Disorders and Stroke; QS, Queen Square; MD, Movement Disorder

substantially by using a prospective validation approach with postmortem confirmation, as demonstrated for the DLB criteria.

Additional investigations have received increasing attention in attempts to improve the poor diagnostic sensitivity at first neurological consultation. Most of the reports on autonomic function testing, cerebrospinal fluid analysis, transcranial sonography, structural and functional neuroimaging, and neurophysiological and neuropsychological testing have been performed in AP patients with clinically established disease. Whether these additional investigations are helpful in patients with suspected early AP is uncertain. Thus, except for MSA, PDD, and DLB, current diagnostic criteria do not include additional testing.

References

1. Litvan I, Bhatia KP, Burn DJ, et al. Movement Disorders Society Scientific Issues Committee report: SIC Task Force appraisal of clinical diagnostic criteria for Parkinsonian disorders. *Mov Disord* 2003; **18**(5): 467–86.

2. Hughes AJ, Daniel SE, Blankson S, et al. A clinicopathologic study of 100 cases of Parkinson's disease. *Arch Neurol* 1993; **50**(2): 140–8.

3. Wenning GK, Ben-Shlomo Y, Hughes A, et al. What clinical features are most useful to distinguish definite multiple system atrophy from Parkinson's disease? *J Neurol Neurosurg Psychiatry* 2000; **68**(4): 434–40.

4. Wenning GK, Ben-Shlomo Y, Magalhães M, et al. Clinicopathological study of 35 cases of multiple system atrophy. *J Neurol Neurosurg Psychiatry* 1995; **58**(2): 160–6.

5. Seppi K, Wenning GK, Jellinger K, et al. Disease progression of dementia with Lewy bodies: a clinicopathological study. *Neurology* 2000; **54**(Suppl 3): S64.002

6. Litvan I, Mangone CA, McKee A, et al. Natural history of progressive supranuclear palsy (Steele–Richardson–Olszewski syndrome) and clinical predictors of survival: a clinicopathological study. *J Neurol Neurosurg Psychiatry* 1996; **60**(6): 615–20.

7. Wenning GK, Litvan I, Jankovic J, et al. Natural history and survival of 14 patients with corticobasal degeneration confirmed at postmortem examination. *J Neurol Neurosurg Psychiatry* 1998; **64**(2): 184–9.

8. Dejerine J, Thomas A. L'atrophie olivo-pontocerebelleuse. *Nouvelle iconographie de la Salpetriere: Clinique des malacies du systeme nerveux* 1900; **13**: 330–70.

9. Shy GM, Drager GA. A neurological syndrome associated with orthostatic hypotension: a clinical-pathologic study. *Arch Neurol* 1960; **2**: 511–27.

10. Adams MR, Van Bogaert L, van der Eecken H. Nigro-striate and cerebello-nigro-striate degeneration. Clinical uniqueness and pathological variability of presenile degeneration of the extrapyramidal rigidity type. *Psychiatr Neurol (Basel)* 1961; **142**: 219–59.

11. Graham JG, Oppenheimer DR. Orthostatic hypotension and nicotine sensitivity in a case of multiple system atrophy. *J Neurol Neurosurg Psychiatry* 1969; **32**(1): 28–34.

12. Papp MI, Kahn JE, Lantos PL. Glial cytoplasmic inclusions in the CNS of patients with multiple system atrophy (striatonigral degeneration, olivopontocerebellar atrophy and Shy–Drager syndrome). *J Neurol Sci* 1989; **94**(1–3): 79–100.

13. Quinn N. Multiple system atrophy – the nature of the beast. *J Neurol Neurosurg Psychiatry* Suppl 1989; 78–89.

14. Spillantini MG, Crowther RA, Jakes R, et al. Filamentous alpha-synuclein inclusions link multiple system atrophy with Parkinson's disease and dementia with Lewy bodies. *Neurosci Lett* 1998; **251**(3): 205–8.

15. Gilman S, Low P, Quinn N, et al. Consensus statement on the diagnosis of multiple system atrophy. *Clin Auton Res* 1998; **8**: 359–62.

16. Wenning GK, Tison F, Seppi K, et al. Development and validation of the Unified Multiple System Atrophy Rating Scale (UMSARS). *Mov Disord* 2004; **19**(12): 1391–402.

17. Stefanova N, Tison F, Reindl M, et al. Animal models of multiple system atrophy. *Trends Neurosci* 2005; **28**(9): 501–6.

18. Gilman S, Wenning GK, Low PA, et al. Second consensus statement on the diagnosis of multiple system atrophy. *Neurology* 2008; **71**(9): 670–6.

19. Scholz SW, Houlden H, Schulte C, et al. SNCA variants are associated with increased risk for multiple system atrophy. *Ann Neurol* 2009; **65**(5): 610–14.

20. Bensimon G, Ludolph A, Agid Y, et al. Riluzole treatment, survival and diagnostic criteria in Parkinson plus disorders: the NNIPPS study. *Brain* 2009; **132**(Pt 1): 156–71.

21. Okazaki H, Lipkin LE, Aronson SM. Diffuse intracytoplasmic ganglionic inclusions (Lewy type) associated with progressive dementia and quadriparesis in flexion. *J Neuropathol Exp Neurol* 1961; **20**: 237–44.

22. Hansen L, Salmon D, Galasko D, et al. The Lewy body variant of Alzheimer's disease: a clinical and pathologic entity. *Neurology* 1990; **40**(1): 1–8.

23. Kosaka K. Dementia and neuropathology in Lewy body disease. *Adv Neurol* 1993; **60**: 456–63.

24. McKeith IG, Galasko D, Kosaka K, et al. Consensus guidelines for the clinical and pathologic diagnosis of dementia with Lewy bodies (DLB): report of the consortium on DLB international workshop. *Neurology* 1996; **47**(5): 1113–24.

25. Takeda A, Mallory M, Sundsmo M, et al. Abnormal accumulation of NACP/alpha-synuclein in neurodegenerative disorders. *Am J Pathol* 1998; **152**(2): 367–72.

26. Muenter MD, Forno LS, Hornykiewicz O, et al. Hereditary form of parkinsonism-dementia. *Ann Neurol* 1998; **43**(6): 768–81.

27. McKeith I, Del Ser T, Spano P, et al. Efficacy of rivastigmine in dementia with Lewy bodies: a randomised, double-blind, placebo-controlled international study. *Lancet* 2000; **356**(9247): 2031–6.

28. Zimprich A, Biskup S, Leitner P, et al. Mutations in LRRK2 cause autosomal-dominant parkinsonism with pleomorphic pathology. *Neuron* 2004; **44**(4): 601–7.

29. Emre M, Aarsland D, Albanese A, et al. Rivastigmine for dementia associated with Parkinson's disease. *N Engl J Med* 2004; **351**(24): 2509–18.

30. McKeith IG, Dickson DW, Lowe J, et al. Diagnosis and management of dementia with Lewy bodies: third report of the DLB Consortium. *Neurology* 2005; **65** (12): 1863–72.

30a. McKeith IG, Ballard, CG, Perry RH, et al. Prospective validation of consensus criteria for the diagnosis of dementia with Lewy bodies. *Neurology* 2000; **10**: 50–8.

31. Goker-Alpan O, Giasson BI, Eblan MJ, et al. Glucocerebrosidase mutations are an important risk factor for Lewy body disorders. *Neurology* 2006; **67**(5): 908–10.

32. Emre M, Aarsland D, Brown R, et al. Clinical diagnostic criteria for dementia associated with Parkinson's disease. *Mov Disord* 2007; **22**(12): 1689–707.

33. Steele JC, Richardson JC, Olszewski J. Progressive Supranuclear Palsy. A heterogeneous degeneration involving the brain stem, basal ganglia and cerebellum with vertical gaze and pseudobulbar palsy, nuchal dystonia and dementia. *Arch Neurol* 1964; **10**: 333–59.

34. Pollock NJ, Mirra SS, Binder LI, et al. Filamentous aggregates in Pick's disease, progressive supranuclear palsy, and

Alzheimer's disease share antigenic determinants with microtubule-associated protein, tau. *Lancet* 1986; **2**(8517): 1211.

35. Imai H, Narabayashi H, Sakata E. "Pure akinesia" and the later added supranuclear ophthalmoplegia. *Adv Neurol* 1987; **45**: 207–12.

36. Lees AJ. The Steele–Richardson–Olszewski syndrome (progressive supranuclear palsy). In: Marsden CD, Fahn S, eds. *Movement disorders 2*. London: Butterworths, 1987; 272–87.

37. Litvan I, Agid Y, Calne D, et al. Clinical research criteria for the diagnosis of progressive supranuclear palsy (Steele–Richardson–Olszewski syndrome): report of the NINDS–SPSP international workshop. *Neurology* 1996; **47**(1): 1–9.

38. Mailliot C, Sergeant N, Bussière T, et al. Phosphorylation of specific sets of tau isoforms reflects different neurofibrillary degeneration processes. *FEBS Lett* 1998; **433**(3): 201–4.

39. Caparros-Lefebvre D, Elbaz A. Possible relation of atypical parkinsonism in the French West Indies with consumption of tropical plants: a case-control study. Caribbean Parkinsonism Study Group. *Lancet* 1999; **354**(9175): 281–6.

40. Houlden H, Baker M, Morris HR, et al. Corticobasal degeneration and progressive supranuclear palsy share a common tau haplotype. *Neurology* 2001; **56**(12): 1702–6.

41. Williams DR, de Silva R, Paviour DC, et al. Characteristics of two distinct clinical phenotypes in pathologically proven progressive supranuclear palsy: Richardson's syndrome and PSP-parkinsonism. *Brain* 2005; **128**: 1247–58.

42. Rebeiz JJ, Kolodny EH, Richardson EP Jr. Corticodentatonigral degeneration with neuronal achromasia. *Arch Neurol* 1968; **18**(1): 20–33.

43. Riley DE, Lang AE, Lewis A, et al. Cortical-basal ganglionic degeneration. *Neurology* 1990; **40**(8): 1203–12.

44. Lang AE, Bergeron C, Pollanen MS, et al. Parietal Pick's disease mimicking cortical-basal ganglionic degeneration. *Neurology* 1994; **44**(8): 1436–40.

45. Kertesz A, Davidson W, Munoz DG. Clinical and pathological overlap between frontotemporal dementia, primary progressive aphasia and corticobasal

degeneration: The Pick complex. *Dement Geriatr Cogn Disord* 1999; **10** (Suppl 1): 46–9.

46. Dickson DW, Bergeron C, Chin SS, et al. Office of Rare Diseases neuropathologic criteria for corticobasal degeneration. *J Neuropathol Exp Neurol* 2002; **61**(11): 935–46.

47. Quinn N. Parkinsonism – recognition and differential diagnosis. *BMJ* 1995; **310**(6977): 447–52.

48. Osaki Y, Ben Shlomo Y, Less AJ, et al. Accuracy of clinical diagnosis of progressive supranuclear palsy. *Mov Disord* 2004; **19**: 181–9.

49. Hughes AJ, Daniel SE, Ben-Shlomo Y, et al. The accuracy of diagnosis of parkinsonian syndromes in a specialist movement disorder sevice. *Brain* 2002; **125**: 861–70.

50. Osaki Y, Ben-Shlomo Y, Lees AJ, et al. A validation exercise on the new consensus criteria for multiple system atrophy. *Mov Disord* 2009; **24**(15):2272–6.

51. Litvan I, MacIntyre A, Goetz CG, et al. Accuracy of the clinical diagnoses of Lewy body disease, Parkinson disease, and dementia with Lewy bodies: a clinicopathologic study. *Arch Neurol* 1998; **55**(7): 969–78.

Parkinson's disease and the spectrum of Lewy body disease

Paolo Barone, Maria Teresa Pellecchia, Marianna Amboni

History

Parkinson's disease (PD) and dementia with Lewy bodies (DLB) are two common presentations of a single, underlying disease process that is thought to be related to the dysregulation of the synaptic protein α-synuclein [1]. It is proposed that PD, PD with dementia (PDD), and DLB represent different manifestations of a continuous disease spectrum of Lewy body disease [1].

Friedrich Heinrich Lewy was the first person to detail the pathological anatomy of PD by personally examining 85 patients [2]. He first described the intraneuronal inclusions, subsequently coined "Lewy bodies" (LBs), in the substantia nigra of PD patients in the early 1900s [3], but he did not attribute an important role to the presence of inclusion bodies for the postmortem diagnosis [4]. The importance of these inclusions, to which Lewy's name was first ascribed by Tretiakoff (Corps de Lewy) in 1919, was seen only after Lewy's death, when LBs began to be considered the defining neuropathological feature of PD. Diffuse Lewy body disease or dementia was identified much later, after the first report of LBs in the cerebral cortex in patients with dementia in 1961 [5]. Ubiquitin and α-synuclein immunocytochemistry in the 1990s allowed easier recognition of LBs [6,7].

The terminology used in the characterization of Lewy body disease (LBD) and clinical syndromes associated with LBD continually evolved. LBD is a term that was proposed in 1984 by Kosaka and colleagues who had been studying the neuropathological changes in patients with dementia for a decade and had examined a series of cases with a combination of LBs in the brainstem, diencephalon, anterior cingulum, amygdala, and cerebral cortex [1]. Kosaka distinguished diffuse LBD with a high LB burden in most areas from brainstem predominant LBD, and transitional LBD that was intermediate between diffuse and brainstem predominant LBD. Clinically, the patients ranged from typical idiopathic PD through cases with parkinsonism and dementia, to a few cases with dementia but no extrapyramidal features [8]. Most experts used the term LBD to refer to the histopathological disorder, but other diagnostic terms included diffuse LBD, cortical LBD, LB dementia, and the LB variant of Alzheimer's disease (AD). The overlap in the clinical and pathological terms generated much confusion. Consensus criteria for the clinical and neuropathological diagnoses were published in 1996 by the Consortium on Dementia with Lewy Bodies [9], which suggested that the clinical syndrome should be termed "DLB," and the neuropathological disorder be termed "LBD." Debate continued on how to label patients with typical features of PD subsequently developing dementia. Most authors apply the label DLB to all patients who develop

Handbook of Atypical Parkinsonism, eds. Carlo Colosimo, David E. Riley, and Gregor K. Wenning. Published by Cambridge University Press. © Cambridge University Press 2011.

parkinsonism after the onset of dementia and also to those who develop dementia within one year from the onset of parkinsonism. The term PDD refers those patients who develop dementia more than one year after the onset of parkinsonism. The recent recognition that dementia becomes increasingly prevalent in PD patients followed over the course of the disease, with a prevalence of up to 78% over eight years [10], prompted the generation of evidence-based criteria for PDD. According to these recently published clinical diagnostic criteria, the term PDD should be used to describe dementia that occurs in the context of well-established PD [11]. However, DLB and PDD share many pathological and clinical features and probably represent two clinical entities on a spectrum of LBD, as underpinned by abnormalities in α-synuclein metabolism [12]. A unitary approach to classification may be preferable for molecular and genetic studies and for developing therapeutics, but the one-year rule should remain in place in research studies in which a distinction needs to be made between DLB and PDD [13]. Given the biological similarities between DLB and PDD, yet variability and differences in clinical presentation, the DLB/PDD Working Group recently agreed to endorse the term "Lewy body disorders" as the umbrella term for PD, PDD, and DLB and to use the term "Lewy body dementias" to refer to PDD and DLB [14].

Clinical findings

Neuroepidemiological studies show that DLB, after AD, is the second most common form of degenerative dementia in older people, responsible for 22% of all cases of dementia [15]. A recent systematic review reported that the prevalence of DLB is 0–5% in the general population [16]. DLB usually presents in late adulthood, between the ages of 60 and 90 years, with no significant gender or ethnic differences in prevalence [9]. The disease is a dementing disorder, and progressive and disabling cognitive impairment is the central feature. Patients show a combination of cortical and subcortical cognitive impairments with significant attentional deficits, in addition to executive and visuospatial dysfunctions. Problems with performing sequential tasks, for example using remote controls, moving in familiar surroundings, and ordering from a menu, are typical symptoms [17]. Patients tend to perform poorly on attention, learning, and constructional praxis. In addition to cognitive impairment, the clinical features of DLB include neuropsychiatric features, motor dysfunction, sleep disorders, and autonomic dysfunction.

The diagnosis of DLB is primarily clinical, with no definitive laboratory or diagnostic testing available. The diagnostic criteria for DLB first published in 1996 by the Consortium on DLB were updated in 2005 [13]. The revised criteria divide clinical features into four categories: central, core, suggestive, and supportive.

Central feature

The central feature, essential for a diagnosis of possible or probable DLB, is a dementia defined as a progressive cognitive decline of sufficient magnitude to interfere with normal social or occupational function. Early memory loss may be absent, whereas deficits in attention, executive function, and visuospatial ability are especially prominent.

Core features

Core features include fluctuating cognition, recurrent visual hallucinations, and spontaneous parkinsonism. Fluctuations refer to periods of time when cognition and arousal are clearly abnormal compared with other periods with normal or near-normal functioning [17].

Table 2.1 Consensus criteria for DLB

Central feature (essential for a diagnosis of possible or probable DLB)
Dementia defined as progressive cognitive decline of sufficient magnitude to interfere with normal social or occupational function; prominent or persistent memory impairment may not necessarily occur in the early stages but is usually evident with progression; deficits on tests of attention, executive function, and visuospatial ability may be especially prominent
Core features (two core features are sufficient for a diagnosis of probable DLB, one for possible DLB)
Fluctuating cognition with pronounced variations in attention and alertness
Recurrent visual hallucinations that are typically formed and detailed
Spontaneous features of parkinsonism
Suggestive features (one or more of these in the presence of one or more core features is sufficient for a diagnosis of probable DLB; in the absence of any core features, one or more suggestive features is sufficient for possible DLB)
REM sleep behavior disorder
Severe neuroleptic sensitivity
Low dopamine transporter uptake in basal ganglia demonstrated by SPECT or PET imaging
Supportive features (commonly present but not proven to have diagnostic specificity)
Repeated falls and syncope
Transient, unexplained loss of consciousness
Severe autonomic dysfunction, e.g. orthostatic hypotension, urinary incontinence
Hallucinations in other modalities
Systematized delusions
Depression
Relative preservation of medial temporal lobe structures on CT/MRI scan
Reduced occipital activity on SPECT/PET perfusion scan
Low-uptake MIBG myocardial scintigraphy
Prominent slow wave activity on EEG with temporal lobe transient sharp waves

Modified from McKeith *et al.* [13]

Fluctuations in alertness and attention may last minutes, hours, or days and, when present, are highly suggestive of DLB. The evaluation of cognitive fluctuations may be difficult in the clinical practice. At least one formal measure of fluctuation, such as the Clinician Assessment of Fluctuation scale [18], the One-Day Fluctuation Assessment Scale [18], or the Mayo Fluctuations Composite Scale [19], needs to be used when applying DLB diagnostic criteria. Recurrent, complex, visual hallucinations are generally present early in the course of the disease and remain one of the most useful clinical markers for a diagnosis of DLB. They are present in 33% of patients at the time of presentation and occur at some point in the course of the disease in 46% of cases [12]. In most patients, hallucinations initially occur during nocturnal hours, but over time they tend to occur also during the day independently of the intensity of the ambient light. The perceived images are usually insects, animals, or people, and these images are so vivid that patients often cannot be convinced that the images are not truly present [17]. Affective responses to the hallucinations vary from indifference to amusement or fear.

Parkinsonism is observed in 75–92% of DLB cases and DLB patients presenting with parkinsonism are, on average, younger than patients presenting with neuropsychiatric features (60 vs. 71 yr) [20,21]. All the manifestations of typical PD may occur, although tremor tends to be more symmetrical and related to posture or action. The severity of extrapyramidal symptoms in DLB is generally similar to that of age-matched PD patients, with or without dementia, with a greater postural instability and gait difficulty in DLB than in non-demented PD patients [22]. As a sign of motor dysfunction, myoclonus may also occur, which may cause confusion with Creutzfeldt–Jakob disease.

Suggestive features

Suggestive features include REM sleep behavior disorder, neuroleptic sensitivity, and low dopamine transporter uptake in basal ganglia. The presence of one or more suggestive features with one or more core features is necessary for a probable diagnosis of DLB. REM sleep behavior disorder (RBD), a parasomnia manifesting by vivid dream enacting behavior, occurs in about 50% of patients with DLB and typically precedes cognitive symptoms by years or even decades [23]. Associated sleep disorders include insomnia, excessive daytime drowsiness, restless legs syndrome, and confusion on waking. Neuroleptic sensitivity to D2-receptor blocking agents is suggestive of DLB and is characterized by the acute onset or exacerbation of parkinsonism and impaired consciousness; however, approximately 50% of patients with DLB receiving typical or atypical antipsychotic drugs do not present this reaction. These agents should never be used as a clinical challenge for diagnosing DLB because of the high morbidity and mortality associated with neuroleptic sensitivity [24].

Supportive features

Supportive features, often present but not proven to be specific for DLB, are autonomic dysfunction, repeated falls and syncope, transient loss of consciousness, non-visual hallucinations, depression, delusions, absence of medial temporal lobe atrophy on CT/MRI scans, abnormal metaiodobenzylguanidine (MIBG) myocardial scintigraphy, and slow wave activity on EEG with temporal lobe transient sharp waves.

Severe autonomic dysfunction may occur early in the disease, featuring orthostatic hypotension, urinary incontinence, constipation, impotence, and swallowing difficulties, and contributing to repeated falls, syncope, and transient losses of consciousness that can be observed in some patients [25]. Falls, often resulting in injury, occur at some point of the disease in 37% of DLB patients [26]. They have been associated with parkinsonism, orthostatic hypotension, vasovagal syncope, and carotid sinus hypersensitivity. Paranoid delusions of persecution, theft, and spousal infidelity occur with some frequency as well and often coexist with hallucinations [27]. Delusions and hallucinations often trigger behavioral problems, leading to profound caregiver distress and precipitating early nursing home admission. Depression is also common in DLB and may appear years before the onset of dementia [27]. Other neuropsychiatric features include anxiety, hallucinations in other sensory modalities (auditory, tactile, and olfactory), aggressivity, agitation, and hypomania.

Overlapping symptoms across the Lewy body disorders

DLB often presents with non-motor symptoms including cognitive impairment, autonomic dysfunction, and psychiatric symptoms. In the early disease stages, this can lead to diagnostic confusion with AD, other autonomic failure syndromes, or primary psychiatric disorders. On the other hand, autonomic and cognitive dysfunctions have been reported in all stages of PD. Constipation may manifest before the classical motor symptoms in about 50% of PD patients [28], and isolated autonomic failure may be the presenting clinical picture of PD [29]. In a prospective study, patients with erectile dysfunction have been reported to have a significantly increased risk of developing PD during the follow-up compared with patients without erectile dysfunction [30]. Bladder and erectile dysfunction, and orthostatic hypotension (OH) may be early findings in PD [31,32], and OH is found in 50% of PDD patients [33].

Cognitive deficits, particularly frontal executive dysfunction and visuospatial deficits, are almost universally identified even in early PD [34]. Community-based studies have suggested that 30–40% of patients with PD will develop clinically defined dementia (PDD). Dementia usually occurs late in the course of PD, an observation proposed by Braak *et al.* [35] that would be in line with the progressive spread of LB pathology from the medulla and olfactory bulb through the pons, midbrain, and basal forebrain, finally to involve cortical areas. However, this theory does not account for DLB cases, 25% of which will never show extrapyramidal features, nor does it account for those patients who develop dementia early in the course of PD [1].

By the end stage, DLB and PDD are often clinically indistinguishable with a combination of extrapyramidal features, cognitive impairment, and psychiatric and autonomic dysfunction. In fact, other than temporal differences in the emergence of symptoms, age at onset, and possibly levodopa responsivity, no major differences between DLB and PDD have been found in any variable examined including cognitive profile, attentional impairment, neuropsychiatric features, sleep disorders, autonomic dysfunction, type and severity of parkinsonism, and responsiveness to cholinesterase inhibitors [13]. The previously mentioned studies confirm the overlap between the key syndromes within the spectrum of LB disorders. The presence and distribution of LB may account for clinically distinct syndromes showing various combinations of parkinsonism, dementia, and autonomic failure [36].

Natural history

Definitive information on the prognosis of patients with DLB is not yet available. Some studies show that patients with DLB experience a cognitive decline similar to that in patients with AD [37,38]. Others suggest a worse prognosis for patients with DLB [39]. Symptom progression occurs in both diseases over time, with an average survival of 7.3 years in DLB (vs. 8.5 yr in AD). Women with DLB seem to have a shorter survival time following dementia onset than men with DLB (6.6 vs. 8.1 yr). Patients with DLB have an increased risk of mortality versus patients with AD, possibly owing to the progression of non-cognitive symptoms [38]. Extrapyramidal signs are strong predictors of mortality and long-term care placement, whereas depressive symptoms are important predictors of long-term care placement and survival in nursing homes. Rest tremor seems to be a protective factor in survival analyses, suggesting that tremor-predominant forms of DLB, which are rare, may have a better prognosis than rigid-predominant forms, similarly to the different forms of PD [38].

DLB patients with established parkinsonism have an annual increase in severity, assessed with the Unified Parkinson's Disease Rating Scale (UPDRS), of 9%, a rate of progression comparable with PD [40]. Progression, comparably with PD, is more rapid in DLB patients with early parkinsonism (49% increase in the motor UPDRS score in one year).

Among neuropsychiatric symptoms, visual hallucinations were significantly more likely to be persistent in DLB as compared to AD [41]. Delusions and auditory hallucinations, which were more frequent at baseline in DLB than in AD, persisted after one year of follow-up in about 40% of patients with DLB and AD.

Laboratory investigations

There are not yet genotypic, serum, or cerebrospinal fluid (CSF) markers to support a diagnosis of DLB. Studies based on CSF have reported interesting preliminary findings for the combination of amyloid β isoforms as well as α-synuclein, and there are interesting results emerging from studies applying proteomic techniques [42]. These findings deserve further investigations to identify reliable biomarkers for DLB.

Functional imaging of the dopamine transporter by SPECT or PET scans can help in the differential diagnosis of probable DLB and AD. Indeed, striatal dopamine transporter (DAT) uptake is low in DLB, owing to the loss of presynaptic dopaminergic terminals, whereas it is normal in AD. Moreover, imaging of DAT may be useful in diagnostically uncertain cases, as an abnormal scan in a patient with possible DLB is strongly suggestive of DLB, according to the revised criteria [43]. It is important to emphasize that DLB patients can have a highly abnormal DAT uptake even in the absence of signs of parkinsonism. In a recent multi-European phase III trial involving 94 probable DLB and 91 probable AD patients, ^{123}I-FP-CIT SPECT correctly identified 78% of DLB and 93% of AD cases diagnosed according to clinical criteria [44]. A similar accuracy (88% sensitivity, 100% specificity) of ^{123}I-FP-CIT SPECT in the diagnosis of DLB has been reported in prospective studies with neuropathological confirmation (Figure 2.1) [45] .

Cardiac scintigraphy with ^{123}I-MIBG provides information on the integrity of the cardiac postganglionic sympathetic neurons. As these autonomic fibers are markedly decreased because of Lewy body-type degeneration in the cardiac plexus, ^{123}I-MIBG scintigraphy shows a low uptake in DLB, irrespective of the presence or absence of clinical

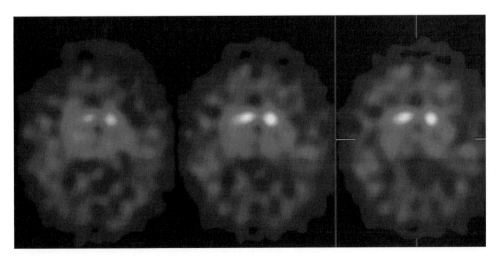

Figure 2.1 Functional imaging of the dopamine transporter by ^{123}I-FP-CIT SPECT showing reduced striatal uptake in a patient affected by dementia with Lewy bodies. (Courtesy: Drs Andrea Varrone and Sabina Pappatà, Institute of Biostructure and Bioimaging, CNR, Naples.) (See color plate section.)

autonomic symptoms. This technique seems to have a high accuracy in the differential diagnosis from AD, where there is no such degeneration [46], and in the early identification of DLB from other neurodegenerative diseases with cognitive impairment [47]. In this regard, ^{123}I-MIBG cardiac scintigraphy showed a sensitivity of 94% and a specificity of 96% for the diagnosis of DLB [47]. It is important to be aware that cardiac impairment owing to other etiologies, such as ischemic heart disease, cardiomyopathy, and diabetes, can also damage the post-ganglionic sympathetic neurons, which may give rise to reduced uptake of myocardial ^{123}I-MIBG.

Other imaging techniques can also be helpful. Brain MRI usually shows relative preservation of the hippocampus and medial temporal lobe, a finding that may help to distinguish DLB from AD [48]. Moreover, MRI shows atrophy of the putamen in DLB, but not in AD [49].

Fluorodeoxyglucose (FDG)-PET and SPECT studies using blood flow markers typically show occipital hypometabolism [50,51] and hypoperfusion [52,53] in DLB. Reductions in parietal glucose metabolism and parietal hypoperfusion have also been shown in DLB patients by PET or SPECT studies [53,54]. Generally, FDG-PET metabolic imaging has shown greater ability to differentiate DLB from non-DLB dementia as compared to SPECT perfusion techniques. On the basis of occipital hypometabolism, discriminant analytical techniques applied to group comparative studies have noted sensitivities of 86–92% for DLB with specificities versus 80–92% for AD [51,55]. However, there is limited evidence of the ability of these techniques to categorize individual patients correctly.

The standard EEG is diffusely abnormal in 90% of DLB patients, showing early slowing of the dominant rhythm and transient temporal slow (4–7 Hz) wave activity [56]. Several studies, based on a small number of patients, have shown more slowing of EEG rhythm in DLB than in AD. It is not possible to differentiate DLB and AD on the basis of EEG [57]. However, a recent study showed relevant group differences in EEGs from posterior derivations between AD and DLB patients, both at early stages and two-year follow-up, suggesting that EEG recordings may act to support discrimination between these two disorders at the earliest stages of dementia [58].

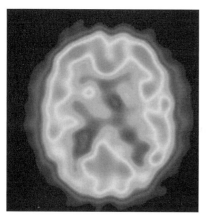 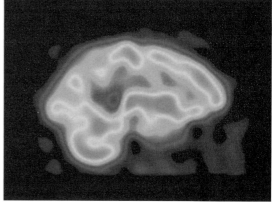

Figure 2.2 FGD-PET showing parietal and occipital hypometabolism in a patient affected by dementia with Lewy bodies. (Courtesy: Drs Andrea Varrone and Sabina Pappatà, Institute of Biostructure and Bioimaging, CNR, Naples.) (See color plate section.)

Genetics

DLB occurs as a sporadic disease in most cases but a number of familial forms have been reported, suggesting the role of genetics [59,60]. Genetic determinants of DLB are heterogeneous and overlap substantially with those of PD.

Alpha-synuclein (SNCA) point mutations [61–63] and whole gene multiplications [64,65] have been associated with clinical and pathological phenotypes ranging from PD to PDD and DLB, highlighting the direct role of α-synuclein overexpression in the pathogenesis of the spectrum of Lewy body disorders. Furthermore, it appears to be a dose effect, with SNCA duplications more often associated with classic PD [66,67] and SNCA triplications more often responsible for PDD and DLB [64,65]. The type of missense mutations might also be critical for the resulting phenotype; in fact the missense mutation A30P is found in association with typical PD [68], whereas E46K and A53T are associated with the entire range of Lewy body disorders [61–63,69]. Alpha-synuclein is a member of a family of pre-synaptic proteins that includes β- and γ-synuclein. There is evidence that β-synuclein might protect against α-synuclein aggregation [70]; therefore, β-synuclein (SNCB) mutations might be responsible for LB disorders. Although SNCB mutations have not been identified in PD patients, two missense mutations (V70M and P123H) have been identified recently in two unrelated DLB index cases [71]. The two mutant β-synuclein proteins have been found to enhance lysosomal pathology in a cell model of synucleinopathy, supporting a causative role for the mutated variants in inducing neurodegeneration [72].

Mutations in the leucine-rich repeat kinase 2 (LRRK2) gene have been identified in familial parkinsonism [73,74]. To date, a wide clinical–pathological spectrum is associated with LRRK2 mutations, which would seem to include clinically and pathologically defined DLB [74,75].

Mutations in the glucocerebrosidase (GBA) gene have been reported in association with parkinsonism and LB pathology among Gaucher's disease patients and their relatives [76–78]. An association between GBA missense mutations and PD has been detected among Ashkenazi Jews [79,80]. More recently, a high prevalence of GBA mutations was reported among patients with pathologically defined DLB [81]. In a case-control study, the frequency of GBA mutations was similar in PD (2.9%) and DLB (3.5%) and significantly higher than the control (0.4%), suggesting a modest population-attributable risk for GBA mutations in Lewy body disorders [82]. Further studies are required to better understand the role of GBA in Lewy body disorders.

Recently, a novel locus for a familial, autosomal dominant DLB has been identified on the long arm of chromosome 2 (2q35-q36; logarithm of odds score of 3.01) in a large Belgian family [83]. Interestingly, this locus for DLB overlaps with PARK11, a locus previously identified in families with autosomal dominant PD [84].

In conclusion, genes involved in genetic forms of PD (SNCA, LRRK2, and GBA) account for most familial DLB cases. Nevertheless, these genes explain only a minority of cases and the discovery of further genes for Lewy body disorders remains a key research priority.

Pathology

Alpha-synuclein represents the common biochemical substrate of pathology in PD, PDD, and DLB [85]. Lewy-related pathology includes LB and Lewy neurites (LNs), which are defined as α-synuclein-positive inclusions in the neuronal cell body and the dendrites and axons, respectively. Alpha-synuclein-positive inclusions have also been found in the pre-synaptic terminals [86] and the glia [87,88].

There are few neuropathological studies directly comparing the three diseases. In PD, LBs and LNs are located mainly in the substantia nigra and other brainstem nuclei such as the locus ceruleus and raphe [89], whereas in DLB, Lewy-related pathology is present in both the brainstem and in a number of cortical areas [90,91]. In PDD, diffuse cortical LBs are the main substrate of dementia [91,92]. Furthermore, senile plaques and neurofibrillay tangles, a hallmark of AD pathology, are common pathological features in both PDD and DLB [91,92]. Some studies have suggested that patients with DLB have more cortical LB load and more brain atrophy compared with PDD patients [93,94]. A more comprehensive report has confirmed greater cortical LB pathology and more senile plaques in DLB versus PDD and has shown that neurofibrillary tangles were rare in both diseases [95].

According to the revised consensus criteria [13], two major aspects have to be considered in the pathological features of DLB. First, because the pattern of regional involvement is more important than total LB count, DLB cases are divided into brainstem predominant, limbic/transitional, and diffuse neocortical subtypes. Second, based on the evidence of the significant concurrent AD pathology [96], it has to be taken into account that "a DLB clinical syndrome is directly related to the severity of Lewy-related pathology and inversely related to the severity of concurrent AD-related pathology" [13].

To date, the complex interaction between LB and AD pathology remains unclear. Some studies have suggested that the process of LB formations is triggered, at least in part, by AD pathology [97,98]. Others have reported that amyloid rather then tau enhances α-synuclein pathology [99]. These intriguing interactions might represent the biomolecular mechanisms underlying the overlapping pathology of DLB and AD [100].

Neuropathological studies have tried to determine whether PDD and DLB are distinct entities or part of a continuum. There is a clear relationship between PDD and DLB with a gradation of neuropathological and neurochemical characteristics across a spectrum spanning from late PDD (parkinsonism for >9.5 years prior to dementia) to early PDD

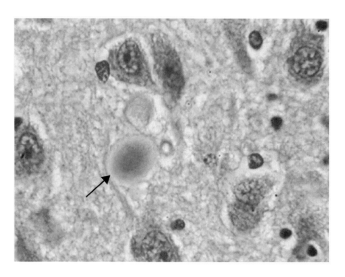

Figure 2.3 Brain cells containing a Lewy body (arrow) (hematoxylin-eosin staining; high-power magnification). (Courtesy: National Human Genome Research Institute.)

(parkinsonism for <9.5 years prior to dementia) and DLB [101]. In particular, a correlation has been found between a longer duration of parkinsonism prior to dementia and less severe cortical LB pathology and fewer senile plaques. The progressive spread of Lewy body pathology as proposed by Braak *et al.* [35], beginning from the medulla and olfactory bulb and advancing through the pons, midbrain, and limbic structures to finally involve the neocortex, is compatible with the observation that dementia usually occurs late in the course of PD. However, this model does not seem applicable for DLB, which starts in the amygdala, advances to the limbic cortex, and finally spreads to the neocortex [102], suggesting that the site of the initial lesions differs in the two diseases.

This apparent inconsistency might be explained by the exclusion of DLB patients in the original Braak analysis [1,14]. Alternatively, it has been proposed that distinct patterns of Lewy-related pathology in PDD and DLB may reflect the regional differences in both dysfunctional neurons and increased expression of α-synuclein protein [103], rather than a caudal-to-rostral-wide spread over the course of the time [104]. This view is supported by the uncertain pathophysiological significance of LBs. The Braak scheme assumes that Lewy pathology reliably identifies dysfunctional neurons, but the assumption that α-synuclein immunopathology detects where PD begins is now debated [104]. In fact, intraneuronal increase of α-synuclein has been identified in several injury models and has been proposed to play a protective role [105–107].

Based on this growing body of evidence, a critical re-evaluation of the Braak staging model is needed to account for the different pathological patterns observed across the Lewy body disorders spectrum.

Management

To date, no therapy altering α-synuclein pathophysiology has been identified. Although α-synuclein-positive LBs are the prominent pathological change in PD, PDD, and DLB, there is a suggestion that amyloid, tau, and α-synuclein pathology may be synergistic, raising the possibility that treatments aimed to affect these abnormal proteins in one disease may be helpful in others as well [108]. On the other hand, there is a symptomatic therapy for the various clinical manifestations of LB disorders. Clinical management includes early detection, diagnosis, and treatment of cognitive impairment; assessment and management of neuropsychiatric and behavioral symptoms; treatment of movement disorder; and management of autonomic dysfunction and sleep disorders [109].

Treatment of cognitive impairment

Cognitive and functional abilities can improve with cholinesterase inhibitor therapy in both PDD and DLB. The cholinesterase inhibitors used in clinical practice include donepezil, rivastigmine, and galantamine. Rivastigmine is the only drug in this class that has been proven to be effective and safe in DLB in a double-blind placebo-controlled trial [110], but open trials on small series have also suggested some efficacy of other cholinesterase inhibitors.

Until not long ago, most published trials in PDD had an open-label design [111,112], except some double-blind studies on donepezil in small series of PDD patients [113,114]. Recently, a large placebo-controlled trial of rivastigmine has reported significant improvement of cognition in PDD [115]. This improvement appeared to be sustained in patients who were able to tolerate an open-label extension [116]. Memantine seems to improve cognitive and neuropsychiatric symptoms in DLB patients, as recently reported [117,118].

Treatment of neuropsychiatric features

Visual hallucinations are often the most troubling neuropsychiatric feature in DLB and PDD, but they do not always require drug treatment. Cholinesterase inhibitors and atypical antipsychotics can be considered for management of hallucinations, delusions, and apathy [110,119–122]. The preferred atypical antipsychotics are clozapine [123–125] and quetiapine [124,126]. Because neuroleptic sensitivity can occur in DLB patients with exposure to even small doses of typical neuroleptics, these agents are strongly discouraged now [127].

Depression is very common in DLB and PDD and sometimes requires treatment. To date, there have been no systematic studies of antidepressive drugs in DLB and PDD depression. However, SSRIs (selective serotonin re-uptake inhibitors) and SNRIs (selective noradrenaline [norepinephrine] re-uptake inhibitors) represent the preferred pharmacological treatment. In fact, the anticholinergic effects of tricyclic antidepressants and paroxetine make these drugs unattractive in the treatment of DLB and PDD.

Treatment of motor dysfunction

Because motor impairment is significant in patients with PDD and in some patients with DLB, studies aimed to treat parkinsonism are relevant. One study has shown that patients with PDD and DLB respond to dopaminergic therapy to a lesser degree than patients without dementia [128].

Recently, L-dopa has been shown to be well tolerated in most DLB patients, but only a third of them experienced significant improvement in parkinsonism [129]. Cognitive functions and neuropsychiatric symptoms were not adversely affected by L-dopa treatment in an open-label study in a small sample of DLB patients [130].

Treatment of other symptoms

Orthostatic hypotension is a crucial and disturbing symptom in patients with LB disorders. Elevating the head of the bed to avoid pressure natriuresis; increasing fluid intake as well as salt in the diet; and using salt tablets, thigh-high compression stockings, fludrocortisone, and midodrine are all potential treatments for OH.

REM sleep behavior disorder is common among patients with Lewy body disorder and responds to clonazepam, usually effective at 0.25–1.0 mg/night [131,132]; to melatonin, usually effective at 3–12 mg/night, either as monotherapy or in association with clonazepam [133]; or to quetiapine, usually effective at 25–100 mg/night [131,132].

Conclusions

The relationship between PDD and DLB is still a matter of intense discussion and debate. Two models have been proposed to explain the link between PDD and LBD: a model whereby there is a PDD–DLB continuum, the boundaries of which are related to the time interval between the onset of cognitive with respect to motor symptoms, and a model where PDD and DLB are defined as discrete entities [13]. The concept that these two disorders have to be viewed as a single entity (α-synucleinopathy) is preferable in order to better research and understand biological and pathophysiological mechanisms and to develop treatment strategies [14]. The genetic determinants of DLB and PDD as well as PD, including alterations in SNCA and LRRK2 and certainly other genes, will offer further insights into the pathogenesis

[17]. Clinical research will help to detect early markers of disease; to better define its natural history; and to develop cognitive and non-cognitive measures, which will be useful in the setting of PDD/DLB. The obvious hope is that disease–modifying or preventing agents can be developed in the near future.

References

1. McKeith IG. Dementia with Lewy bodies and Parkinson's disease with dementia: where two worlds collide. *Pract Neurol* 2007; 7: 374–82.

2. Holdorff B. Friedreich Heinrich Lewy (1885–1950) and his work. *J Hist Neurosci* 2002; 11: 19–28.

3. Lewy FH. Paralysis agitans I Pathologische Anatomie. In: Lewandowsky M, ed. Handbuch der Neurologie. Vol III. Berlin: Springer, 1912; 920–33.

4. Lewy FH. Historical introduction: The basal ganglia and their disease. *Trans Am Neurol Assoc* 1942; 20: 1–20.

5. Okazaki H, Lipkin L, Aronson S. Diffuse intracytoplasmic ganglionic inclusions (Lewy type) associated with progressive dementia and quadriparesis. *J Neuropathol Exp Neurol* 1961; 20: 237–44.

6. Dickson DW. Tau and synuclein and their role in neuropathology. *Brain Pathol* 1999; 9: 657–61.

7. Kosaka K. Dementia and neuropathology in Lewy body disease. *Adv Neurol* 1993; 60: 456–63.

8. Kosaka K, Yoshimura M, Ikeda K, et al. Diffuse type of Lewy body disease: progressive dementia with abundant cortical Lewy bodies and senile changes of varying degree – a new disease? *Clin Neuropathol* 1984; 3(5): 185–92.

9. McKeith IG, Galasko D, Kosaka K, et al. Consensus guidelines for the clinical and pathologic diagnosis of dementia with Lewy bodies (DLB): report of the consortium on DLB workshop. *Neurology* 1996; 47: 1113–24.

10. Aarsland D, Anderson K, Larsen JP, et al. Prevalence and characteristics of dementia in Parkinson disease: an 8-year prospective study. Arch Neurol 2003; 60: 387–392.

11. Emre M, Aarsland D, Brown R , et al. Clinical diagnostic criteria for dementia associated with Parkinson's disease. *Mov Disord* 2007; 22(12): 1689–707.

12. McKeith IG, Burn D. Spectrum of Parkinson's disease, Parkinson's dementia and Lewy body dementia. In: DeKosky ST, ed. *Neurologic Clinics*. WB Saunders: Philadelphia, 2000; 865–83.

13. McKeith, Dickson DW, Lowe J, et al. Diagnosis and management of dementia with Lewy bodies. Third report of the DLB consortium. *Neurology* 2005; 65: 1863–72.

14. Lippa CF, Duda JE, Grossman M, et al. DLB and PDD boundary issues. Diagnosis, treatment, molecular pathology, and biomarkers. *Neurology* 2007; 68: 812–19.

15. Rahkonen T, Eloniemi-Sulkava U, Rissanen S, et al. Dementia with Lewy bodies according to the consensus criteria in a general population aged 75 years or older. *J Neurol Neurosurg Psychiatry* 2003; 74: 720–4.

16. Zaccai J, McCracken C, Brayne C. A systematic review of prevalence and incidence studies of dementia with Lewy bodies. *Age Ageing* 2005; 34: 561–6.

17. Boeve BF. Clinical, diagnostic, genetic and management issues in dementia with Lewy bodies. *Clin Sci* 2005; 109: 343–54.

18. Walker MP, Ayre GA, Cummings JL, et al. The Clinician Assessment of Fluctuation and the One Day Fluctuation Assessment Scale. Two methods to assess fluctuating confusion in dementia. *Br J Psychiatry* 2000; 177: 252–6.

19. Ferman TJ, Smith GE, Boeve BF, et al. DLB fluctuations: specific features that reliably differentiate from AD and normal aging. *Neurology* 2004; 62: 252–6.

20. Geldmacher DS. Dementia with Lewy bodies: diagnosis and clinical approach. *Cleve Clin J Med* 2004; 71: 789–800.

21. Del Ser T, McKeith IG, Anand R, et al. Dementia with Lewy bodies: findings from an international multicentre study. *Int J Geriatr Psychiatry* 2001; 15: 1034–45.

22. Burn DJ, Rowan EN, Minett T, et al. Extrapyramidal features in Parkinson's disease with and without dementia and

dementia with Lewy bodies: a cross-sectional comparative study. *Mov Disord* 2003; **18**: 884–9.

23. Ferman TJ, Boeve, BF, Smith GF, et al. Dementia with Lewy bodies may present as dementia and REM sleep behaviour disorder without parkinsonism or hallucinations. *J Int Neuropsychol Soc* 2002; **8**: 907–14.

24. Geser F, Wenning GK, Poewe W, et al. How to diagnose dementia with Lewy bodies: state of the art. *Mov Disord* 2005; **20**(Suppl 12): 11–20.

25. Horimoto Y, Matsumoto M, Akatsu H, et al. Autonomic dysfunctions in dementia with Lewy bodies. *J Neurol* 2003; **250**: 530–3.

26. Ballard CG, Shaw F, Lowery K, et al. The prevalence, assessment and associations of falls in dementia with Lewy bodies and Alzheimer's disease. *Dement Geriatr Cogn Disord* 1999; **10**: 97–103.

27. Aarsland D, Ballard C, Larsen J, et al. A comparative study of psychiatric symptoms in dementia with Lewy bodies and Parkinson's disease with and without dementia. *Int J Geriatr Psychiatry* 2001; **16**: 528–36.

28. Korczyn AD. Autonomic nervous system disturbances in Parkinson's disease. *Adv Neurol* 1990; **53**: 463–8.

29. Kaufmann H, Nahm K, Purohit D, et al. Autonomic failure as the initial presentation of Parkinson's disease and dementia with Lewy bodies. *Neurology* 2004; **28**: 1093–5.

30. Gao X, Chen H, Schwarzschild MA, et al. Erectile dysfunction and the risk of Parkinson's disease. *Am J Epidemiol* 2007; **166**: 1446–50.

31. Chaudhuri KR, Naidu Y. Early Parkinson's disease and non-motor issues. *J Neurol* 2008; **255**(Suppl 5): 33–8.

32. Goldstein DS. Orthostatic hypotension as an early finding in Parkinson's disease. *Clin Auton Res* 2006; **16**: 46–54.

33. Peralta C, Stamfer M, Karner E, et al. Orthostatic hypotension and attention in Lewy body disorders. *Mov Disord* 2004; **19**: S331–2.

34. Lees AJ, Smith E. Cognitive deficits in Parkinson's disease. *Brain* 1983; **106**: 257–70.

35. Braak H, Del Tredici K, Rub U, et al. Staging of brain pathology related to sporadic Parkinson's disease. *Neurobiol Aging* 2003; **24**: 197–211.

36. Poewe W. Dysautonomia and cognitive dysfunction in Parkinson's disease. *Mov Disord* 2005; (Suppl 17): 374–78.

37. Ballard CG, O'Brien J, Morris CM, et al. The progression of cognitive impairment in dementia with Lewy bodies. *Int J Geriatr Psychiatry* 2001; **16**: 499–503.

38. Williams MM, Xiong C, Morris JC, et al. Survival and mortality differences between dementia with Lewy bodies vs Alzheimer disease. *Neurology* 2006; **67**: 1935–41.

39. Neef D, Walling AD. Dementia with Lewy bodies vs Alzheimer's disease. Tips from other journals. *Am Fam Physician* 2006; **73**: 1223–9.

40. Ballard CG, McKeith IG, Swann A, et al. One year follow-up of parkinsonism in dementia with Lewy bodies. *Dement Geriatr Cogn Disord* 2000; **11**: 219–22.

41. Ballard CG, O'Brien JT, Swann AG, et al. The natural history of psychosis and depression in dementia with Lewy bodies and Alzheimer's disease: persistence and new cases over 1 year of follow-up. *J Clin Psychiatry* 2001; **62**: 46–9.

42. Aarsland D, Kurz M, Beyer M, et al. Early discriminatory diagnosis of dementia with Lewy bodies. *Dement Geriatr Cogn Disord* 2008; **25**: 195–205.

43. O'Brien JT, McKeith IG, Walker Z, et al. Diagnostic accuracy of 123I-FP-CIT SPECT in possible dementia with Lewy bodies. *Br J Psychiatry* 2009; **194**: 34–9.

44. McKeith I, O'Brien J, Walker Z, et al. Sensitivity and specificity of dopaminergic transporter imaging with 123I-FP-CIT SPECT in dementia with Lewy bodies; a phase III multi-centre, prospective study. *Lancet Neurol* 2007; **6**: 305–13.

45. Walker Z, Jaros E, Walker RW, et al. Dementia with Lewy bodies: a comparison of clinical diagnosis, FP-CIT single photon emission computed tomography imaging and autopsy. *J Neurol Neurosurg Psychiatry* 2007; **78**: 1176–81.

46. Taki J, Yoshita M, Tamada M, et al. Significance of I-123-metaiodobenzylguanidine scintigraphy as a pathophysiological indicator in the assessment of Parkinson's disease and related movement disorders: It can be a specific marker for Lewy body disease. *Ann Nucl Med* 2004; **18**: 453–61.

47. Estorch M, Camacho V, Paredes P, et al. Cardiac 123I-metaiodobenzylguanidine imaging allows early identification of dementia with Lewy bodies during life. *Eur J Nucl Med Mol Imaging* 2008; **35**: 1636–41.

48. Burton EJ, Barber R, Mukaetova-Ladinska EB, et al. Medial temporal lobe atrophy on MRI differentiates Alzheimer's disease from dementia with Lewy bodies and vascular cognitive impairment: a prospective study with pathological verification of diagnosis. *Brain* 2009; 132(1): 195–203.

49. Cousins DA, Burton EJ, Burn D, et al. Atrophy of the putamen in dementia with Lewy bodies but not Alzheimer's disease. *Neurology* 2003; **61**: 1191–5.

50. Albin RL, Minoshima S, Damato CJ, et al. Fluoro-deoxyglucose positron emission tomography in diffuse Lewy body disease. *Neurology* 1996; **47**: 462–6.

51. Minoshima S, Foster NL, Sima AAF, et al. Alzheimer's disease versus dementia with Lewy bodies: cerebral metabolic distinction with autopsy confirmation. *Ann Neurol* 2001; **50**: 358–65.

52. Colloby SJ, Fenwick JD, Williams ED, et al. A comparison of 99Tc-HMPAO SPECT changes in dementia with Lewy bodies and Alzheimer's disease using statistical parametric mapping. *Eur J Nucl Med* 2002; **29**: 615–22.

53. Lobotesis K, Fenwick JD, Phipps A, et al. Occipital hypoperfusion on SPECT in dementia with Lewy bodies but not AD. *Neurology* 2001; **56**: 643–9.

54. Kemp PM, Holmes C. Imaging in dementia with Lewy bodies: a review. *Nucl Med Commun* 2007; **28**: 451–6.

55. Ishii K, Imamwa T, Sasaki M, et al. Regional cerebral glucose metabolism in dementia with Lewy bodies and Alzheimer's disease. *Neurology* 1998; **51**: 125–30.

56. Briel RC, McKeith IG, Barker WA, et al. EEG findings in dementia with Lewy bodies and Alzheimer's disease. *J Neurol Neurosurg Psychiatry* 1999; **66**: 401–3.

57. Barber PA, Varma AR. Lloyd JJ, et al. The electroencephalogram in dementia with Lewy bodies. *Acta Neurol Scand* 2000; **101**: 53–6.

58. Bonanni L, Thomas A, Tiraboschi P, et al. EEG comparisons in early Alzheimer's disease, dementia with Lewy bodies and Parkinson's disease with dementia patients with a 2-year follow-up. *Brain* 2008; **131**(3): 690–705.

59. Harding AJ, Das A, Kril JJ, et al. Identification of families with cortical Lewy body disease. *Am J Med Genet B Neuropsychiatr Genet* 2004; **28**: 118–22.

60. Tsuang DW, Di Giacomo L, Bird TD. Familial occurrence of dementia with Lewy bodies. *Am J Geriatr Psychiatry* 2004; **12**: 179–88.

61. Morfis L, Cordato DJ. Dementia with Lewy bodies in an elderly Greek male due to alpha-synuclein gene mutation. *J Clin Neurosci* 2006; **13**: 942–4.

62. Yamaguchi K, Cochran EJ, Murrell JR, et al. Abundant neuritic inclusions and microvacuolar changes in a case of diffuse Lewy body disease with the A53T mutation in the alpha-synuclein gene. *Acta Neuropathol* 2005; **110**: 298–305.

63. Zarranz JJ, Alegre J, Gomez-Esteban JC, et al. The new mutation, E46K, of alpha-synuclein causes Parkinson and Lewy body dementia. *Ann Neurol* 2004; **55**: 164–73.

64. Fuchs J, Nilsson C, Kachergus J, et al. Phenotypic variation in a large Swedish pedigree due to SNCA duplication and triplication. *Neurology* 2007; **68**: 916–22.

65. Singleton AB, Farrer M, Johnson J, et al. α-Synuclein locus triplication causes Parkinson's disease. *Science* 2003; **302**: 841.

66. Chartier-Harlin MC, Kachergus J, Roumier C, et al. Alpha-synuclein locus duplication as a cause of familial Parkinson's disease. *Lancet* 2004; **364**: 1167–9.

67. Ibanez P, Bonnet AM, Debarges B, et al. Causal relation between alpha-synuclein gene duplication and familial Parkinson's disease. *Lancet* 2004; **364**: 1169–71.

68. Kruger R, Kuhn W, Leenders KL, et al. Familial parkinsonism with synuclein pathology: clinical and PET studies of A30P mutation carriers. *Neurology* 2001; **56**: 1355–62.

69. Golbe LI, Di Iorio G, Sanges G, et al. Clinical genetic analysis of Parkinson's disease in the Contursi kindred. *Ann Neurol* 1996; **40**: 767–75.

70. Hashimoto M, Rockenstein E, Mante M, et al. Beta-synuclein inhibits α-synuclein aggregation: a possible role as an

antiparkinsonian factor. *Neuron* 2001; **32**: 213–23.

71. Ohtake H, Limprasert P, Fan Y, et al. Beta-synuclein gene alterations in dementia with Lewy bodies. *Neurology* 2004; **63**: 805–11.

72. Wei J, Fujita M, Nakai M, et al. Enhanced lysosomal pathology caused by beta-synuclein mutants linked to dementia with Lewy bodies. *J Biol Chem* 2007; **282**: 28904–14.

73. Paisan-Ruiz C, Jain S, Evans EW, et al. Cloning of the gene containing mutations that cause PARK8-linked Parkinson's disease. *Neuron* 2004; **44**: 595–600.

74. Zimprich A, Biskup S, Leitner P, et al. Mutations in LRRK2 cause autosomal-dominant parkinsonism with pleomorphic pathology. *Neuron* 2004; **44**: 601–7.

75. Ross OA, Toft M, Whittle AJ, et al. Lrrk2 and Lewy body disease. *Ann Neurol* 2006; **59**: 388–93.

76. Goker-Alpan O, Schiffmann R, LaMarca ME, et al. Parkinsonism among Gaucher disease carriers. *J Med Genet* 2004; **41**(12): 937–40.

77. Halperin A, Eistein D, Zimran A. Increased incidence of Parkinson disease among relatives of patients with Gaucher disease. *Blood Cells Mol Dis* 2006; **36**(3): 426–8.

78. Tayebi N, Walker J, Stubblefield B, et al. Gaucher disease with parkinsonian manifestations: does glucocerebrosidase deficiency contribute to a vulnerability to parkinsonism? *Mol Genet Metab* 2003; **79**(2): 104–9.

79. Aharon-Peretz J, Rosenbaum H, Gershoni-Baruch R. Mutations in the glucocerebrosidase gene and Parkinson's disease in Ashkenazi Jews. *N Engl J Med* 2004; **351**: 1972–7.

80. Clark LN, Ross BM, Wang Y, et al. Mutations in the glucocerebrosidase gene are associated with early-onset Parkinson disease. *Neurology* 2007; **69**: 1270–7.

81. Goker-Alpan O, Giasson BI, Eblan MJ, et al. Glucocerebrosidase mutations are an important risk factor for Lewy body disorders. *Neurology* 2006; **67**: 908–10.

82. Mata IF, Samii A, Schneer SH, et al. Glucocerebrosidase gene mutations: a risk factor for Lewy body disorders. *Arch Neurol* 2008; **65**(3): 379–82.

83. Bogaerts V, Engelborghs S, Kumar-Singh S, et al. A novel locus for dementia with Lewy bodies: a clinically and genetically heterogeneous disorder. *Brain* 2007; **130**: 2277–91.

84. Pankratz N, Nichols WC, Uniacke SK, et al. Significant linkage of Parkinson disease to chromosome 2q36–37. *Am J Hum Genet* 2003; **72**: 1053–7.

85. Spillantini MG, Schmidt ML, Lee VM, et al. α-Synuclein in Lewy bodies. *Nature* 1997; **388**: 839–40.

86. Kramer ML, Schulz-Schaeffer WJ. Presynaptic α-synuclein aggregates, not Lewy bodies, cause neurodegeneration in dementia with Lewy bodies. *J Neurosci* 2007; **27**: 1405–10.

87. Braak H, Sastre M, Bohl JR, et al. Parkinson's disease: lesions in dorsal horn layer I, involvement of parasympathetic and sympathetic pre- and postganglionic neurons. *Acta Neuropathol* 2007; **113**: 421–9.

88. Piao YS, Mori F, Hayashi S, et al. α-Synuclein pathology affecting Bergmann glia of the cerebellum in patients with α-synucleinopathies. *Acta Neuropathol* 2003; **105**: 403–9.

89. Gelb DJ, Oliver E, Gilman S. Diagnostic criteria for Parkinson disease. *Arch Neurol* 1999; **56**: 33–9.

90. Apaydin H, Ahlskog JE, Parisi JE, et al. Parkinson disease neuropathology: later developing dementia and loss of the levodopa response. *Arch Neurol* 2002; **59**: 102–12.

91. Aarsland D, Perry R, Brown A, et al. Neuropathology of dementia in Parkinson's disease: a prospective, community-based study. *Ann Neurol* 2005; **58**: 773–6.

92. Tsuboi Y, Dickson DW. Dementia with Lewy bodies and Parkinson's disease with dementia: are they different? *Parkinsonism Relat Disord* 2005; **11**(Suppl 1): S47–51.

93. Iseki E. Dementia with Lewy bodies: reclassification of pathological subtypes and boundary with Parkinson's disease or Alzheimer's disease. *Neuropathology* 2004; **24**: 72–8.

94. Richard IH, Papka M, Rubio A, et al. Parkinson's disease and dementia with

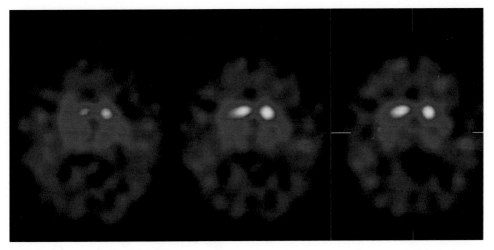

Figure 2.1 Functional imaging of the dopamine transporter by 123I-FP-CIT SPECT showing reduced striatal uptake in a patient affected by dementia with Lewy bodies. (Courtesy: Drs Andrea Varrone and Sabina Pappatà, Institute of Biostructure and Bioimaging, CNR, Naples.)

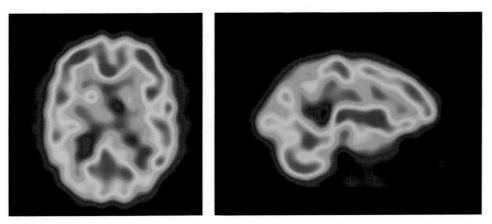

Figure 2.2 FGD-PET showing parietal and occipital hypometabolism in a patient affected by dementia with Lewy bodies. (Courtesy: Drs Andrea Varrone and Sabina Pappatà, Institute of Biostructure and Bioimaging, CNR, Naples.)

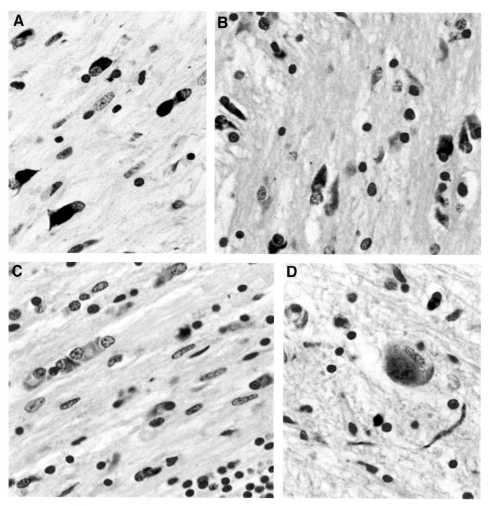

Figure 3.8 Glial cytoplasmic inclusions in multiple system atrophy: (A) in globus pallidus (Gallyas silver impregnation); (B) in pontine base (α-synuclein); (C) in frontal white matter (anti-ubiquitin); (D) neuronal cytoplasmic inclusion and neurites in pontine base (α-synuclein). (400X magnification.)

Lewy bodies: one disease or two? *Mov Disord* 2002; **17**: 1161–5.

95. Harding AJ, Broe GA, Halliday GM. Visual hallucinations in Lewy body disease relate to Lewy bodies in the temporal lobe. *Brain* 2002; **125**: 391–403.

96. Lippa CF, McKeith I. Dementia with Lewy bodies: improving diagnostic criteria. *Neurology* 2003; **60**: 1571–2.

97. Iseki E, Togo T, Susuki K, et al. Dementia with Lewy bodies from the perspective of tauopathy. *Acta Neuropathol* 2003; **105**: 265–70.

98. Marui W, Iseki E, Nakai T, et al. Progression and staging of Lewy pathology in brains from patients with dementia with Lewy bodies. *J Neurol Sci* 2002; **195**: 153–9.

99. Pletnikova O, West N, Lee MK, et al. Abeta deposition is associated with enhanced cortical alpha-synuclein lesions in Lewy body diseases. *Neurobiol Aging* 2005; **26**: 1183–92.

100. Obi K, Akiyama H, Kondo K, et al. Relationship of phosphorylated alpha-synuclein and tau accumulation to Abeta deposition in the cerebral cortex of dementia with Lewy bodies. *Exp Neurol* 2008; **210**: 409–20.

101. Ballard CG, Ziabreva I, Perry R, et al. Differences in neuropathologic characteristic across the Lewy body dementia spectrum. *Neurology* 2006; **67**: 1931–4.

102. Katsuse O, Iseki E, Marui W, et al . Developmental stages of cortical Lewy bodies and their relation to axonal transport blockage in brains of patients with dementia with Lewy bodies. *J Neurol Sci* 2003; **211**: 29–35.

103. Solano SM, Miller DW, Augood SJ, et al. Expression of alpha-synuclein, parkin, and ubiquitin carboxy-terminal hydrolase L1 mRNA in human brain: genes associated with familial Parkinson's disease. *Ann Neurol* 2000; **47**: 201–10.

104. Burke RE, Dauer WT, Vonsattel JP. A critical evaluation of the Braak staging scheme for Parkinson's disease. *Ann Neurol* 2008; **64**(5): 485–91.

105. Kholodilov NG, Neystat M, Oo TF, et al. Increased expression of rat synuclein1 in the substantia nigra pars compacta identified by differential display in a model of developmental target injury. *J Neurochem* 1999; **73**: 2586–99.

106. Manning-Bog AB, McCormack AL, Purisai MG, et al. Alpha-synuclein overexpression protects against paraquat-induced neurodegeneration.*J Neurosci* 2003; **23**: 3095–9.

107. Purisai MG, McCormack AL, Langston WJ, et al. Alpha-synuclein expression in the substantia nigra of MPTP-lesioned non-human primates. *Neurobiol Dis* 2005; **20**: 898–906.

108. Lee VM, Giasson BI, Trojanowski JQ. More than just two peas in a pod: common amyloidogenic properties of tau and alpha-synuclein in neurodegenerative diseases. *Trends Neurosci* 2004; **27**(3): 129–34.

109. Barber R, Panikkar A, McKeith IG. Dementia with Lewy Bodies: diagnosis and management. *Int J Geriatr Psychiatry* 2001; **16**(suppl 1): S12–18.

110. McKeith I, Del Ser T, Spano P, et al. Efficacy of rivastigmine in dementia with Lewy bodies: a randomised, double-blind, placebo-controlled international study. *Lancet* 2000; **356**: 2031–2036.

111. Werber EA, Rabey JM. The beneficial effect of cholinesterase inhibitors on patients suffering from Parkinson's disease and dementia. *J Neural Transm* 2001; **108**(11): 1319–25.

112. Hutchinson M, Fazzini E. Cholinesterase inhibition in Parkinson's disease. *J Neurol Neurosurg Psychiatry* 1996; **61**(3): 324–5.

113. Leroi I, Brandt J, Reich SG, et al. Randomized placebo-controlled trial of donepezil in cognitive impairment in Parkinson's disease. *Int Geriatr Psychiatry* 2004; **19**(1): 1–8.

114. Ravina B, Putt M, Siderowf A, et al. Donepezil for dementia in Parkinson's disease: a randomized, double blind, placebo-controlled, crossover study. *J Neurol Neurosurg Psychiatry* 2005; **76**(7): 934–9.

115. Emre M, Aarsland D, Albanese A, et al. Rivastigmine for dementia associated with Parkinson's disease. *N Eng J Med* 2004; **351**(24): 2509–18.

116. Poewe W, Wolters E, Emre M, et al. Long-term benefits of rivastigmine in dementia associated with Parkinson's disease: an

active treatment extension study. *Mov Disord* 2006; **21**(4): 456–61.

117. Aarsland D, Ballard C, Walker Z, et al. Memantine in patients with Parkinson's disease dementia or dementia with Lewy bodies: a double-blind, placebo-controlled, multicentre trial. *Lancet Neurol* 2009; **8**(7): 613–18.

118. Emre M, Tsolaki M, Bonuccelli U, et al. Memantine for patients with Parkinson's disease dementia or dementia with Lewy bodies: a randomized, double-blind, placebo-controlled trial. *Lancet Neurol* 2010; **9**(10): 969–77.

119. Bergman J, Lerner V. Successful use of donepezil for the treatment of psychotic symptoms in patients with Parkinson's disease. *Clin Neuropharmacol* 2002; **25**(2): 107–10.

120. Bullock R, Cameron A. Rivastigmine for the treatment of dementia and visual hallucinations associated with Parkinson's disease: a case series. *Curr Med Res Opin* 2002; **18**(5): 258–64.

121. Fergusson E, Howard R. Donepezil for the treatment of psychosis in dementia with Lewy bodies. *Int J Geriatr Psychiatry* 2000; **15**: 280–1.

122. Lanctot KL, Herrmann N. Donepezil for behavioural disorders associated with Lewy bodies: a case series. *Int J Geriatr Psychiatry* 2000; **15**: 338–45.

123. Chacko RC, Hurley RA, Harper RG, et al. Clozapine for acute and maintenance treatment of psychosis in Parkinson's disease. *Fall* 1995; **7**(4): 471–5.

124. Dewey RJ, O'Suilleabhain P. Treatment of drug-induced psychosis with quetiapine and clozapine in Parkinson's disease. *Neurology* 2000; **55**: 1753–4.

125. Valldeoriola F, Nobbe FA, Tolosa E. Treatment of behavioural disturbances in Parkinson's disease. *J Neural Transm* 1997; Suppl 51: 175–204.

126. Takahashi H, Yoshida K, Sugita T, et al. Quetiapine treatment of psychotic symptoms and aggressive behavior in patients with dementia with Lewy bodies: a case series. *Prog Neuropsychopharmacol Biol Psychiatry* 2003; **27**: 549–53.

127. McKeith I, Fairbairn A, Perry R, et al. Neuroleptic sensitivity in patients with senile dementia of Lewy body type. *Br Med J* 1992; **305**: 673–8.

128. Bonelli SB, Ransmayr G, Steffelbauer M, et al. L-dopa responsiveness in dementia with Lewy bodies, Parkinson's disease with and without dementia. *Neurology* 2004; **63**(2): 376–8.

129. Molloy S, McKeith I, O'Brien J, et al. The role of levodopa in the management of dementia with Lewy bodies. *J Neurol Neurosurg Psychiatry* 2005; **76**(9): 1200–3.

130. Molloy S, Rowan EN, O'Brien JT, et al. Effect of levodopa on cognitive function in Parkinson's disease with and without dementia and dementia with Lewy bodies. *J Neurol Neurosurg Psychiatry* 2006; **77**: 1323–8.

131. Boeve BF, Silber M, Ferman T. Current management of sleep disturbances in dementia. *Curr Neurol Neurosci Rep* 2001; **2**(2): 169–77.

132. Boeve BF, Silber M, Ferman T. REM sleep behavior disorder in Parkinson's disease and dementia with Lewy bodies. *J. Geriatr Psychiatry Neurol* 2004; **17**: 146–57.

133. Boeve BF, Silber M, Ferman T. Melatonin for treatment of REM sleep behavior disorder in neurologic disorders: results in 14 patients. *Sleep Med* 2003; **4**: 281–4.

Chapter 3

Multiple system atrophy

Roberta Granata and Gregor K. Wenning

Multiple system atrophy (MSA) is a sporadic and rapidly progressive neurodegenerative disorder presenting with autonomic failure combined with levodopa-refractory parkinsonism and/or cerebellar ataxia. In the past years, significant developments have expanded the research field, leading to a more accurate understanding of MSA. Here we review the current views on etiopathogenesis, present the novel clinical diagnostic criteria, and discuss the most recent investigations and treatment strategies including disease-modifying drug trials.

Introduction

Multiple system atrophy is characterized by a variable combination of autonomic failure, poorly levodopa-responsive parkinsonism, cerebellar ataxia, and pyramidal symptoms. Typically, neuronal cell loss in the basal ganglia, cerebellum, pontine and inferior olivary nuclei, pyramidal tract, intermediolateral cell column, and Onuf's nucleus as well as gliosis and α-synuclein-containing glial cytoplasmic inclusions (GCIs) are observed [1].

Until 1969, three cardinal presentations of MSA including striatonigral degeneration (SND), sporadic olivopontocerebellar atrophy (OPCA), and Shy–Drager syndrome (SDS) were regarded as distinct entities until Graham and Oppenheimer recognized their substantial clinicopathological overlap and proposed MSA as an umbrella term [2]. Ubiquitin-positive GCIs were first reported in 1989 [3] and subsequently confirmed as a cellular marker of MSA regardless of the phenotypic presentation. Alpha-synuclein immunostaining of GCIs was first described in the late 1990s. Following this discovery, MSA has been regarded as α-synucleinopathy along with Parkinson's disease (PD), Lewy body dementia (DLB), and pure autonomic failure (PAF). Quinn proposed the first set of diagnostic criteria and distinguished the motor subtypes MSA-P and MSA-C, although there was unintended overlap. Furthermore, he allowed an abnormal external sphincter EMG fiinding as a diagnostic criterion, thereby creating practical difficulties [4]. For these reasons, a consensus conference was convened in 1998 that proposed clinical guidelines exclusively, for the diagnosis of MSA. The latter was divided into MSA-P and MSA-C depending on the predominant motor presentation at the time of examination [5]. Based on improvements of early diagnosis by defining warning signs (red flags) and sensitive neuroimaging indices, the consensus guidelines were revised ten years later [6]. A Unified MSA Rating Scale (UMSARS) quantifying disease severity has been established and validated in the meantime by the European

---

Handbook of Atypical Parkinsonism, eds. Carlo Colosimo, David E. Riley, and Gregor K. Wenning.
Published by Cambridge University Press. © Cambridge University Press 2011.

MSA Study Group (EMSA-SG) [7]. UMSARS has been applied in the EMSA natural study confirming the rapid progression of autonomic failure, cerebellar ataxia, and parkinsonism (Wenning *et al.*, unpublished data). Animal models have become available as preclinical test-beds for translational neuroprotection and neuroregeneration studies [8]. The first clinical trials have been conducted by two independent consortia using minocycline [9] and riluzole [10]. Other international networks have been established in the last few years including NAMSA (North American MSA Study Group) [11], JAMSAC (Japanese MSA Consortium), and CNMSA (Chinese MSA Study Group). Globalization of MSA research has led not only to the aforementioned trial activities but also to the first genetic breakthrough by indentifying variants in the α-synuclein gene and their association with increased disease risk in a large population of MSA patients [12]. In addition, several pedigrees with monogenic MSA, but yet unidentified loci, have been reported [13].

Epidemiology

Multiple system atrophy, in both genders, usually progresses for an average of nine years from the sixth decade until death [14]. There are few epidemiological surveys suggesting that MSA is an orphan disease with a prevalence rate of 4.4/100 000 and an incidence rate of 3/100 000 per year [15,16].

Clinical presentation and diagnosis

Clinically, cardinal features include autonomic failure, parkinsonism, cerebellar ataxia, and pyramidal signs in any combination (Table 3.1). Two major motor presentations can be distinguished. In the western hemisphere, parkinsonian features predominate in 60% of patients (MSA-P subtype), and cerebellar ataxia is the major motor feature in 40% of patients (MSA-C subtype) [17]. The reverse distribution is observed in the eastern hemisphere [18,19]. MSA-associated parkinsonism is dominated by progressive akinesia and rigidity whereas tremor is less common than in PD. Postural stability is compromised early on; however, recurrent falls at disease onset are unusual in contrast to progressive supranuclear palsy (PSP). The cerebellar disorder of MSA is composed of gait ataxia, limb kinetic ataxia, and scanning dysarthria, as well as cerebellar oculomotor disturbances. Dysautonomia develops in almost all patients with MSA [20]. Early impotence (erectile dysfunction) is virtually universal in men, and urinary incontinence or incomplete bladder emptying, often early in the disease course or as presenting symptoms, are frequent. Orthostatic hypotension (OH) is present in two-thirds of patients [17].

The clinical diagnosis of MSA rests largely on history and physical examination. The revised consensus criteria [6] specify three diagnostic categories of increasing certainty: possible, probable, and definite. Whereas a definite diagnosis requires neuropathological evidence of a neuronal multisystem degeneration (SND, OPCA, central autonomic degeneration) and abundant GCIs [21], the diagnosis of possible and probable MSA is based on the presence of clinical and imaging features (Tables 3.2–3.4). In addition, supportive features (warning signs or red flags) as well as non-supportive features may be considered (Figures 3.1–3.5; Tables 3.5 and 3.6).

Natural history and progression

The disease affects men and women alike. It starts in the sixth decade and progresses relentlessly until death, on average nine years after disease onset [10,14,22]. There is a considerable variation of disease duration with survival times of up to 15 years or more. Predictors of poor

Table 3.1 Clinical presentation of multiple system atrophy according to the EMSA-Registry

437 patients (53% male; mean age at disease onset 58 years; mean disease duration 5.8 years; 68% MSA-P; 32% MSA-C)

Autonomic failure

- Urinary symptoms (83%)
  - urge incontinence (73%)
  - incomplete bladder emptying (48%)
  - erectile failure (84%)
- Orthostatic hypotension (75%; syncope 19%)
- Chronic constipation (33%)

Parkinsonism

  - bradykinesia and rigidity (93%)
  - postural instability (89%)
  - rest tremor (33%)
  - freezing of gait (38%)

Cerebellar ataxia

  - gait ataxia (86%)
  - limb ataxia (78%)
  - ataxic dysarthria (69%)

Pyramidal signs

- Babinski sign (28%)
- Generalized hyperreflexia (43%)

Neuropsychiatric features

- Depression (41%)
- Hallucinations (5.5%)
- Dementia (4.5%)
- Insomnia (19%)
- Daytime sleepiness (17%)
- Restless legs (10%)

Modified according to Koellensperger *et al.* [17]

Table 3.2 Consensus criteria for the diagnosis of probable multiple system atrophy

A sporadic, progressive, adult (>30 yr)-onset disease characterized by

- Autonomic failure involving urinary incontinence (inability to control the release of urine from the bladder, with erectile dysfunction in males) or an orthostatic decrease of blood pressure within 3 min of standing by at least 30 mmHg systolic or 15 mmHg diastolic blood pressure

and

- Poorly levodopa-responsive parkinsonism (bradykinesia with rigidity, tremor, or postural instability)

or

- A cerebellar syndrome (gait ataxia with cerebellar dysarthria, limb ataxia, or cerebellar oculomotor dysfunction)

Table 3.3 Consensus criteria for the diagnosis of possible multiple system atrophy

A sporadic, progressive, adult (>30 yr)-onset disease characterized by

- Parkinsonism (bradykinesia with rigidity, tremor, or postural instability)

or

- A cerebellar syndrome (gait ataxia with cerebellar dysarthria, limb ataxia, or cerebellar oculomotor dysfunction)

and

- At least one feature suggesting autonomic dysfunction (otherwise unexplained urinary urgency, frequency or incomplete bladder emptying, erectile dysfunction in males, or significant orthostatic blood pressure decline that does not meet the level required in probable MSA)

and

- At least one of the additional features shown in Table 3.4

Table 3.4 Additional features of possible multiple system atrophy

Possible MSA-P or MSA-C

- Babinski sign with hyperreflexia
- Stridor

Possible MSA-P

- Rapidly progressive parkinsonism
- Poor response to levodopa
- Postural instability within 3 yr of motor onset
- Gait ataxia, cerebellar dysarthria, limb ataxia, or cerebellar oculomotor dysfunction
- Dysphagia within 5 yr of motor onset
- Atrophy on MRI of putamen, middle cerebellar peduncle, pons, or cerebellum
- Hypometabolism on FDG-PET in putamen, brainstem, or cerebellum

Possible MSA-C

- Parkinsonism (bradykinesia and rigidity)
- Atrophy on MRI of putamen, middle cerebellar peduncle, or pons
- Hypometabolism on FDG-PET in putamen
- Presynaptic nigrostriatal dopaminergic denervation on SPECT or PET

outcome include female gender, older age at onset, autonomic failure, and rapid progression [23]. The motor variants of MSA are associated with similar survival [24], although disease progression is more rapid in MSA-P than in MSA-C patients [18]. Most MSA-P patients succumb to sudden death reflecting loss of serotonergic neurons in the ventrolateral medulla [25]. Other causes of death may include aspiration pneumonia or pulmonary embolism.

The recent natural history study by EMSA-SG applied the UMSARS [7] and confirmed rapid progression with an average increase of UMSARS I scores (reflecting activities of daily living) by 16.8% in the first six months compared to baseline. Furthermore, UMSARS II (motor examination) scores increased by 26.1% and UMSARS IV (global disability) scores by 12.5% [26] (Figure 3.6).

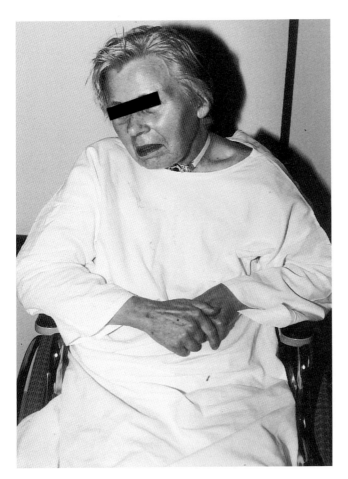

Figure 3.1 Patient with multiple system atrophy of the parkinsonian type showing non-L-Dopa responsive akinetic-rigid parkinsonism and early development of the "wheelchair sign." In addition, the patient showed a disproportionate antecollis and a pronounced inspiratory stridor that caused respiratory failure leading to tracheostomy. [Reproduced with permission from reference 194.]

Investigations

The diagnosis of MSA rests on both history and neurological examination. Additional investigations may be performed according to the consensus criteria. These include cardio-vascular autonomic function tests, external sphincter EMG, and neuroimaging. However, previous studies have been conducted largely in patients with advanced MSA and therefore the diagnostic validity of additional testing in early MSA remains to be determined.

Autonomic function tests

Demonstration of severe autonomic failure in the early disease stages supports a presumptive diagnosis of MSA although the specificity of such findings has not been investigated to date. Abnormal results of autonomic function tests (AFTs) may be associated with a plethora of symptoms that impair quality of life and warrant therapeutic intervention [27]. If left untreated, overt OH may result in cognitive decline and recurrent falls. Furthermore, untreated urinary retention may lead to urinary tract infections and urosepsis ultimately.

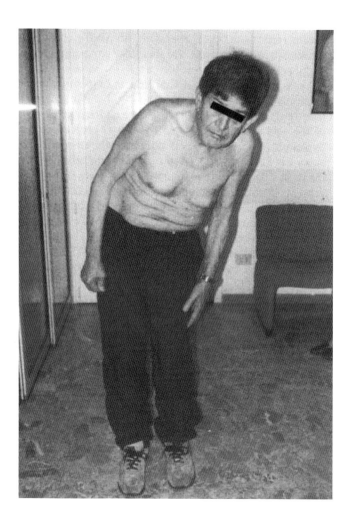

Figure 3.2 Pisa syndrome in a patient with multiple system atrophy. [Reproduced with permission from reference 195.]

Cardiovascular autonomic function tests

Symptoms of OH such as postural dizziness, neck or "coat hanger" ache, and visual disturbances should be investigated further by determining the presence and degree of blood pressure drop on standing. In patients with severe motor disability, tilt table testing is a valuable alternative. According to international practice, OH is defined as systolic blood pressure drop of at least 20 mmHg and/or as diastolic pressure drop of at least 10 mmHg within three minutes of standing or tilt typically associated with an insufficient rise in heart rate. The consensus criteria for MSA require a more severe degree of OH for a diagnosis of probable MSA (see previous sections). Recent evidence suggests that delayed OH beyond three minutes of postural challenge may occur in up to 50% of patients with orthostatic symptoms [28]. Therefore, extended postural challenge up to ten minutes may be justified in patients with suspected MSA and symptoms of orthostatic intolerance. Cardiovascular autonomic failure in MSA primarily reflects degeneration of central autonomic pathways with failure of the baroreflex whereas idiopathic PD (IPD) is characterized by Lewy body deposition in cardiac sympathetic ganglia and the enteric plexus. Reflecting these differences in pathology, cardiovascular autonomic function tests in a dedicated unit can distinguish MSA from IPD

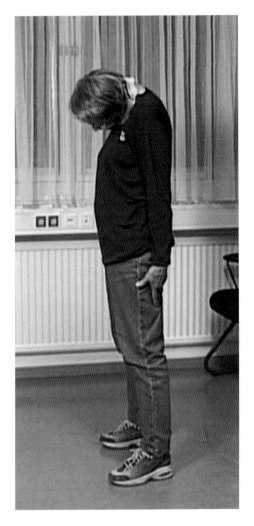

Figure 3.3 Disproportionate antecollis of a patient with multiple system atrophy of the parkinsonian type.

based on the severity, distribution, and pattern of autonomic deficits that may increase during repeated testing [29].

Urological work-up

Investigation of bladder function is obligatory in all patients with suspected MSA [30]. A careful history should be taken to reveal typical symptoms such as urinary urgency, frequency, nocturia, double micturition, retention, and urge incontinence. A severe urge incontinence with or without incomplete bladder emptying is a characteristic feature of MSA and may occur rarely in terminal IPD. Non-neurogenic causes of urological symptoms such as urinary incontinence following transurethral resection of the prostate (TURP) or a descending pelvic floor in multiparous women should be excluded. Urinary tract infection may mimic neurogenic urological failure and requires exclusion. Furthermore, post-void residual volume needs to be determined by ultrasound or if necessary by catheterization.

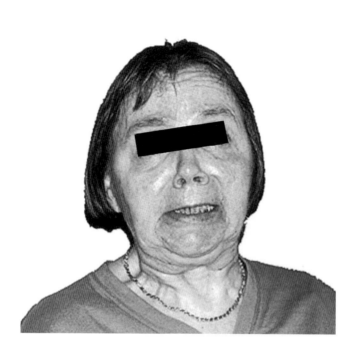

Figure 3.4 *Risus sardonicus* (RS) of a patient with multiple system atrophy of the parkinsonian type. [Reproduced with permission from reference 196.]

Videourodynamic testing shows typical changes in MSA. In the early stages, there is evidence of detrusor hyperreflexia, frequently combined with bladder neck incompetence, reflecting sphincter dysfunction. This constellation of features leads to urinary urgency, frequency, and urge incontinence ultimately. Later, there is loss of detrusor hyperreflexia and bladder atonia ensues with incomplete bladder emptying [31].

Sphincter electromyography

A pathological sphincter EMG showing spontaneous activity, prolonged action potential duration, as well as polyphasia is seen in many patients with probable MSA even if there are no symptoms of urogenital failure [32]. However, the frequency of such abnormalities in the early disease stages is currently unknown. Similar changes may be present in advanced IPD or PSP. False-positive results often result from transabdominal prostatectomy or other surgical procedures in the pelvic floor. Finally, pathological sphincter EMGs are frequent in multiparous women. On the other hand, a neurogenic sphincter EMG discriminates well between the early stages of IPD and MSA-P as well as idiopathic late-onset cerebellar ataxia (ILOCA) and MSA-C [33].

Cerebrospinal fluid investigations

Elevated neurofilament concentrations in CSF have been identified as diagnostic markers of atypical parkinsonism (AP) versus IPD. Both heavy- and light-chain neurofilaments may be increased without significant changes over time [34–37]. However, discrimination of MSA and PSP/corticobasal degeneration (CBD) appears impossible, limiting the utility of CSF testing in clinical practice. Indeed, given the availability of sensitive non-invasive diagnostic tools such as MRI, CSF studies in MSA patients should be limited to scientific protocols.

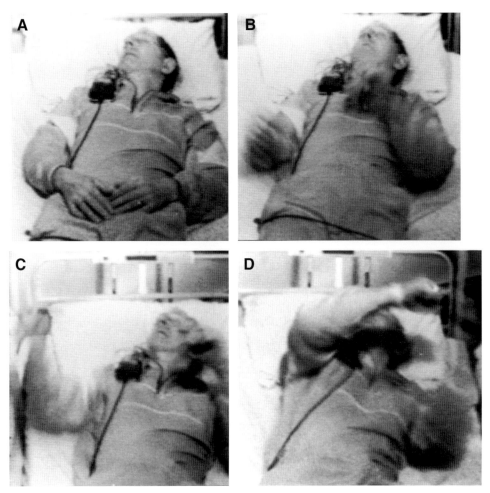

Figure 3.5 REM sleep behavior disorder during polysomnography in a patient with multiple system atrophy of the parkinsonian type. The attacks of sleep behavior disorder were the presenting feature and initially misdiagnosed as epileptic attacks. During the attacks the patient would strike out with his arms, often with sleep talking/shouting and recall of frightening dreams if awakened.

Neuroendocrinological investigations

Impaired stimulation of growth hormone by clonidine or arginine has been reported to discriminate both MSA-P from IPD as well as MSA-C from ILOCA [38,39]. However, clonidine testing has subsequently generated contradictory results whereas arginine testing appears to be more robust [40]. To date, the available diagnostic protocols have not entered routine clinical practice because of their invasive and time-consuming design.

Neuroimaging

Brooks and Seppi have recently reviewed the entire world literature on neuroimaging in MSA [41]. The reader is referred to their extensive reference list for in-depth studies.

Table 3.5 Supportive features (red flags) for a diagnosis of multiple system atrophy

- Orofacial dystonia
- Disproportionate antecollis
- Camptocormia (severe anterior flexion of the spine) and/or Pisa syndrome (severe lateral flexion of the spine)
- Contractures of hands or feet
- Inspiratory sighs
- Severe dysphonia
- Severe dysarthria
- New or increased snoring
- Cold hands and feet
- Pathologic laughter or crying
- Jerky, myoclonic postural/action tremor

Table 3.6 Non-supportive features for a diagnosis of multiple system atrophy

- Classical pill-rolling tremor
- Clinically significant neuropathy
- Hallucinations not induced by drugs
- Onset age after 75 yr
- Family history of ataxia or parkinsonism
- Dementia on (DSM-IV)
- White matter lesions suggesting multiple sclerosis

Modified according to Gilman S *et al.* [6]

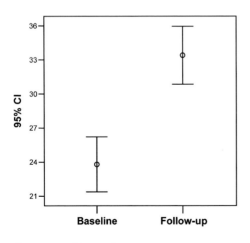

Figure 3.6 Error bars showing narrow confidence intervals with no overlap of UMSARS II both at baseline and 12-months' follow-up visit (n=50) (*p*<0.0001) (modified according to Geser et al. [26]). [Reproduced with permission from reference 26.]

Structural imaging

Transcranial sonography

Transcranial sonography (TCS) may help to diagnose AP by showing normoechogenicity of the substantia nigra, which contrasts with hyperechogenicity in most IPD patients [42].

However, these data have been obtained in clinically definite patients; the predictive value of TCS in the early disease stages remains to be determined. Furthermore, differentiation of MSA and PSP is difficult, based on TCS criteria including third ventricle size and lentiform echogenicity [43]. Finally, the diagnostic yield of TCS depends on a sufficient acoustic temporal bone window.

Cranial computerized tomography

CT can be normal in MSA; however, in about half of the patients there may be atrophy of the brainstem, cerebellum, and rarely cerebral cortex. In general, sensitivity and specificity of CT are fairly low in AP and therefore all patients with suspected MSA should be investigated by 1.5 Tesla MRI (Figure 3.7).

Magnetic resonance tomography

The majority of published MRI studies in MSA patients were conducted with 1.5 Tesla machines [41]. T2-weighted imaging may reveal typical changes such as putaminal hypointensity, periputaminal hyperintensity (rim sign), atrophy of the brainstem and middle cerebellar peduncle, and the hot cross bun sign. [44]. These alterations can differentiate MSA-P from IPD as well as OPCA from other causes of ILOCA. However, the sensitivity is suboptimal (80%) and discrimination of MSA and PSP may not always be possible.

Quantitative planimetric MR-based atrophy indices may contribute to the differentiation of IPD versus MSA-P (atrophic middle cerebellar peduncle in MSA; reduced putaminal volume in MSA-P) and PSP (reduced ratio of midbrain versus pontine area) [45]. However, these findings need to be corroborated. Volumetric studies have also been used to discriminate MSA from other disorders with parkinsonism [46] and to determine rates of brain volume loss over time [47,48]. Pathologically elevated putaminal diffusivity as quantitatively determined by the regional apparent diffusion coefficient (rADC) has been reported as a useful marker of MSA and PSP versus IPD (without discriminating between the two atypical disorders) [49,50]; however, more evidence, particularly in the early disease stages, is required to firmly establish putaminal rADCs as a diagnostic tool in clinical practice. Higher diagnostic yield may be gained by rADCs in the middle cerebllar peduncle and pons, which allow the discrimination of MSA-P from both IPD and PSP [51,52].

Functional neuroimaging

Region of interest-based visualization of presynaptic dopaminergic function by SPECT or PET and appropriate ligands allows the differentiation of degenerative from non-degenerative causes of parkinsonism. Unfortunately, MSA-P cannot reliably be discriminated from other degenerative disorders with parkinsonism using these standard techniques [53]. However, sophisticated analysis of SPECT or PET data using statistical parametric mapping (SPM) has shown a specific dopaminergic denervation of the midbrain in MSA-P versus IPD patients [54]. In addition, demonstration of striatal dopaminergic denervation in patients presenting with ILOCA supports a diagnosis of MSA-C [6]. Striatal dopamine D2-receptor binding can be determined by SPECT or PET and is typically reduced in patients with MSA while IPD patients show normal or increased binding [53]. However, there may be considerable overlap between the patient groups limiting the predictive value of receptor binding. Increased microglial activation has been identified in the basal ganglia and brainstem of MSA patients using PET and C-PK11195 [55]. This finding may

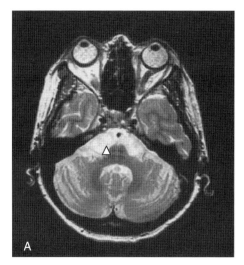 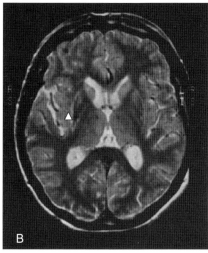

Figure 3.7 Typical findings on routine 1.5 Tesla MRI in a patient with multiple system atrophy: pontine atrophy with hot cross bun sign (A, arrowhead) as well as lateral rim-like hyperintensity along the putamen (rim sign) combined with intraputaminal hypointensity (B, arrowhead). [No copyright permission required.]

represent a useful surrogate marker of disease activity. Its diagnostic utility remains to be determined.

Fluorodeoxyglucose (FDG)–PET typically shows hypometabolism in the striatum, brainstem, and cerebellum of MSA patients [56–58]. This pattern has been confirmed by complex network analysis [59]. FDG–PET, compared to visual analysis, is particularly useful in combination with SPM-based analysis, increasing the sensitivity in the differential diagnosis of disorders with parkinsonism up to 95% [60].

Most IPD patients – even those without overt autonomic symptoms – show a reduced cardiac sympathetic innervation using metaiodobenzylguanidine (MIBG) scintigraphy [61–63] or F-dopamine PET [64] while these investigations are usually normal in MSA and PSP patients. However, some IPD patients may show normal cardiac MIBG uptake [65] whereas sympathetic cardiac denervation can occur in MSA [66] (Gilman, personal communication).

MR-spectroscopy has generated controversial results in studies addressing the differential diagnosis of disorders with parkinsonism and cannot be recommended for routine use [41].

In summary, currently there are no investigations that can prove a diagnosis of MSA. However, there are a number of characteristic findings in patients with clinically probable MSA (Table 3.7). Whether these are predictive in those patients with possible or suspected MSA remains to be investigated in prospective studies, ideally with postmortem validation.

Pathology

Neuropathological changes in the CNS of MSA cases involve different regions including the striatum, substantia nigra pars compacta, locus coeruleus, cerebellum, pontine nuclei, inferior olives, and the intermediolateral columns [67,68]. The selective distribution of neurodegeneration in anatomically related regions suggests a linked degenerative process [69,70]. The two clinical subtypes of MSA, MSA-P and MSA-C, display a predominant albeit

Table 3.7 Additional investigations in multiple system atrophy

Investigation	Typical results
Cardiovascular autonomic function tests	Orthostatic hypotension (≥20/10 mmHg systolic/diastolic blood pressure drop) Impaired reflex tachycardia Impaired heart rate variability Impaired Valsalva maneuver Impaired rise of plasma noradrenaline upon standing
Arginine/clonidine challenge test	Impaired release of growth hormone (controversial)
Thermoregulatory sweat test (TST), quantitative sudomotor axon reflex test (QSART)	Sudomotor dysfunction (an-/hypohidrosis) owing to pre- and postganglionic sympathetic failure
Sympathetic skin response	Abnormal or absent
CSF	Increased neurofilament (light and heavy chain) level
External sphincter EMG	Denervation/reinnervation (nonspecific)
Transcranial sonography	Lentiform hyperechogenicity and nigral normoechogenicity
CT	Unhelpful
MRI (1.5 Tesla)	Basal ganglia abnormalities (putaminal atrophy/hyperintense putaminal rim/putaminal hypointensity), infratentorial signal change (hot cross bun sign), cerebellar and/or brain stem atrophy
MRI (DWI)	Increased diffusivity of putamen (posterior > anterior), rostral pons and middle cerebellar peduncle
MR volumetry	Regional volume loss (putamen in MSA-P, MCP, brainstem and cerebellum in MSA-C)
MIBG scintigraphy	Normal postganglionic sympathetic function (no reduced myocardial MIBG uptake)
FP-CIT SPECT IBZM SPECT F-dopa-PET C-raclopride-PET F-PK11195-PET FDG-PET	Reduced striatal dopamine transporter binding Reduced striatal dopamine D2 receptor binding Reduced striatal F-Dopa uptake Reduced striatal dopamine D2 receptor binding Microglial activation in basal ganglia and brainstem areas Reduced striatal, frontal, and infratentorial metabolism

overlapping pattern of neuropathology, involving the striatonigral system in MSA-P and the olivopontocerebellar system in MSA-C [67,69].

A neuropathology-based grading scale of MSA has been proposed for both striatonigral and olivopontocerebellar lesions. The scale defines four degrees of severity (SND 0-III and OPCA 0-III) and further supports the concept of minimal change MSA to capture subtle neuronal loss and gliosis in vulnerable areas [14,71–73].

More recently, the neuropathology of autonomic failure in MSA has received considerable attention. Lesions of the vagal nucleus and nucleus ambiguus have been characterized [74]. Furthermore, selected medullary, pontomedullary, and pontine nuclei appear to be affected as well [67,75–78]. Cholinergic cell loss at the mesopontine level (pedunculopontine tegmental nuclei/laterodorsal tegmental nuclei involved in the sleep control) has also been reported in MSA [78]. The hypothalamus is affected [79]; in particular, several studies demonstrated a loss of arginine-vasopressin neurons in the posterior portion of the paraventricular nucleus and in the suprachiasmatic nucleus [74], and a loss of hypocretin/orexin neurons of the posterolateral hypothalamus [80]. All these cell populations are involved in circadian regulation of endocrine and autonomic functions. At lower levels of the autonomic nervous system, lesions are observed typically in sympathetic preganglionic neurons in the intermediolateral column of the thoracolumbar spinal cord that have been linked to OH [67,70]. Alpha-synuclein aggregates have also been reported in sympathetic ganglia of MSA brains [81,82]. Urogenital and sexual disorders have been related to neuropathological changes in parasympathetic preganglionic neurons of the spinal cord including Onuf's nucleus [67,83–85].

Some years ago, GCIs containing α-synuclein filaments as well as a range of other cytoskeletal proteins have been defined as a cellular hallmark of MSA [1,3,86–89] (Figure 3.8; Table 3.8). MSA has since been classified as α-synucleinopathy, together with IPD and DLB [90]. On this basis, the second consensus statement on the diagnosis of MSA [6] requires "… evidence of widespread and abundant CNS alpha-synuclein-positive CGIs in association with neurodegenerative changes in striatonigral or olivopontocerebellar systems" for a diagnosis of "definite MSA" [6,21].

Although the localization of GCIs is widespread, they appear more prominent in areas affected by severe neuronal loss and they are also correlated with the severity and duration of the disease [91,92].

In addition, neuronal cytoplasmic inclusions (NCIs) and neuronal nuclear inclusions (NNIs) have been reported in MSA, mainly in the putamen, substantia nigra, inferior olivary nucleus, motor cortex, dentate gyrus, and pontine nuclei [81,93–100]. NCIs, NNIs, and abnormal neurons show no spatial correlation with the CGIs' distribution. In addition, in the minimal change pattern of MSA, CGIs are widely distributed in the brain whereas neuronal loss is confined to substantia nigra (SN) or olivopontocerebellar (OPC) systems. These notions lead to the hypothesis that the primary pathological event takes place in glial cells and that neuronal pathology follows the gliopathy [14,73,91,94,95,101].

Thus, α-synuclein aggregates seem to play a fundamental role in the pathogenesis of MSA, but the underlying mechanism is still incompletely understood. GCI-like inclusions developed in transgenic animals overexpressing α-synuclein in oligodendrocytes, suggesting that abnormal production of α-synuclein may overcome the ability of oligodendrocytes to degrade it [102–105]. However, Miller and coworkers reported that α-synuclein mRNA is not expressed in oligodendrocytes of both normal and MSA human brains, indicating that the α-synuclein accumulation in these cells is ectopic [106].

Early myelin alterations in MSA brains have been demonstrated recently by the presence of altered myelin basic protein and p25α [101]. The p25α protein, also called tubulin polymerization promoting protein (TPPP), has been shown to colocalize with α-synuclein-positive CGIs and to accumulate abnormally in MSA oligodendrocytes [107–110, 113–116]. Transfer of p25α to oligodendroglial cell bodies has been detected in early MSA, suggesting that this event causes myelin damage followed by α-synuclein

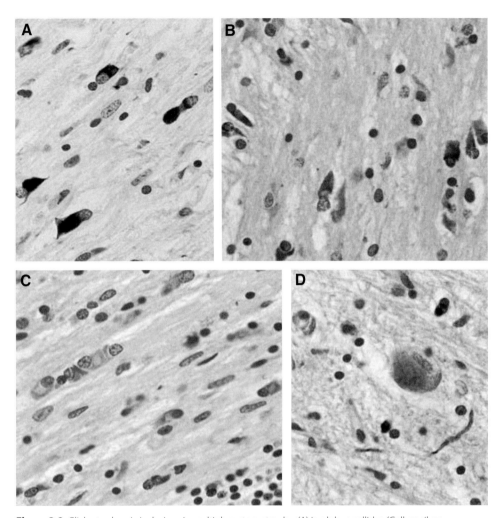

Figure 3.8 Glial cytoplasmic inclusions in multiple system atrophy: (A) in globus pallidus (Gallyas silver impregnation); (B) in pontine base (α-synuclein); (C) in frontal white matter (anti-ubiquitin); (D) neuronal cytoplasmic inclusion and neurites in pontine base (α-synuclein). (400X magnification.) (See color plate section.)

aggregation and secondary neurodegeneration [101,110]. These findings have provided additional evidence to consider MSA as a primary oligodendrogliopathy with GCI accumulation causing oligodendroglia–myelin degeneration [101,111–113]. However, this pathogenic oligodendroglial mechanism may still occur synergistically with a direct neuronal alteration (as in a neuronal synucleinopathy), as both nonfibrillary and fibrillary α-synuclein accumulation seems to be present in neurons albeit more restricted [113,114].

Alpha-synuclein-related lesions have been associated with other neuropathological changes such as neuronal loss, reactive microgliosis, microglial activation, iron deposition, and myelin degeneration [107–109]. In particular, microglial activation suggests that neuroinflammatory mechanisms are also involved in MSA pathogenesis [111,115,116].

Table 3.8 List of protein constituents identified in glial cytoplasmic inclusions from human multiple system atrophy

- α-synuclein
- α-tubulin
- β-tubulin
- 14-3-3 protein
- Bcl-2
- Carbonic anhydrase isoenzyme IIa
- cdk-5 (cyclin-dependent kinase 5)
- Midkine[a]
- DARPP32
- Dorfin
- Heat shock proteins Hsc70 and Hsp70
- Isoform of four-repeat tau protein (hypophosphorylated)
- DJ-1
- Mitogen-activated protein kinase (MAPK)
- NEDD-8
- Other microtubule-associated proteins (MAPs): MAP-1A and -1B; MAP-2 isoform 1, and MAP-2 isoform 4
- Phosphoinositide 3-kinase (PI3K)
- p25 α/TPPP
- Septin -2, -3, -5, -6, and -9
- Transferrin[a]
- Ubiquitin SUMO-1 (small ubiquitin modifier 1)

[a] Known oligodendroglial marker

Etiopathogenesis

Environmental factors

The underlying etiopathogenesis of MSA is still not understood; however, similar to other sporadic neurodegenerative diseases and MSA, a complex interaction of genetic and environmental mechanisms seems likely [117]. However, owing to principal limitations of environmental studies such as recall bias (over-reporting of exposures) and selection bias (patients with severe disease are less able to participate), there are no convincing findings. Mercury, methanol, carbon tetrachloride, carbon disulfide, and cyanide have been associated with MSA-like parkinsonism in a small series of cases [118]. Furthermore, manganese intoxication reported in miners can produce clinical, neuroimaging, and pathological findings that may overlap with those of MSA [118]. The few controlled studies available in the literature have attempted to correlate the increased risk of MSA with occupational and daily habits, such as working exposure to solvents, plastic monomers, additives, metals, various other toxins [5,119,120], and a history of farming [102,121]. However, the increased risk of MSA related to occupational toxins and pesticides has not been confirmed by any recent study [122].

Smoking appears to be a protective factor for MSA as in PD [120,123,124], even if a recent report did not confirm these data [122]. Rigg's hypothesis, according to which a selective survival bias might explain the inverse association between smoking, AD, and PD, because smokers have a higher mortality than non-smokers, seems to be refuted by the presence of inverse smoking habits in MSA and PSP patients [124]. Alcohol consumption showed no association in an earlier study [5] but it was reported to be protective in a more recent one [122].

Genetics

MSA is generally considered a sporadic disease [125]; however, rare familial cases have been reported [125,126]. Recently, Hara *et al.* observed several families with autosomal recessive inheritance as suggested by affected siblings in three of four families [13]. In addition, some studies suggest that spinocerebellar ataxia type 1 (SCA1) and other forms of spinocerebellar ataxias as well as fragile X–associated tremor/ataxia syndrome (FXTAS) may be associated with MSA-like presentations [128–132].

A second genetic approach focused on the α-synuclein gene because of the fundamental role of α-synuclein inclusion pathology in MSA [3,87,101]. All previous studies (including sequencing of the SNCA coding sequence, gene dosage measurements, microsatellite testing, and haplotype studies) failed to identify significant associations of SNCA variants with MSA [133–136]. However, these negative results can be explained by small sample size. Indeed, a recent candidate single nucleotide polymorphism (SNP) genomic study demonstrated that SNCA variants, and particularly its cerebellar variant, play a role in the development of MSA [137,138].

Other genes coding for apolipoprotein E, dopamine β-hydroxylase, ubiquitin C-terminal hydrolase-1, fragile X mental retardation 1, and leucine-rich kinase 2 showed no association with MSA [135].

In contrast, polymorphisms of several genes involved in inflammatory processes have been associated with an elevated MSA risk. These include genes coding for interleukin-1A, interleukin-1B, interleukin-8, intercellular adhesion molecule-1 and tumor necrosis factor, and alpha-1-antichymotrypsin [139–143]. For example, there is a five-fold risk to develop MSA with homozygosity for interleukin-1A allele 2. The alpha-1-antichymotrypsin AA genotype (ACT-AA) is associated with a significantly earlier onset and faster disease progression [140]. A recent study showed that MSA is also associated with polymorphisms of genes involved in oxidative stress [144].

Animal models

In the last decade, several animal models have been developed to support the studies on MSA [8]. Because the etiopathogenesis of the disease remains unknown, the design of MSA animal models has been based on phenotypic replication of core pathological features of the disease, which finally result in specific motor dysfunction. Currently, toxin and transgenic approaches are applied to achieve MSA-like neurodegeneration in rodents. Stereotactic or systemic use of selective neurotoxins, which induce loss of neurons in the substantia nigra pars compacta and loss of medium spiny neurons in the dorsolateral striatum, is a common approach to replicate striatonigral degeneration underlying levodopa-unresponsive parkinsonism of MSA-P [145–149]. In addition, three transgenic mouse models have been developed to study the role of GCI-like pathology [103–105]. In these transgenic mice, selective promoters are used to over-express human α-synuclein targeted in oligodendroglia.

Transgenic MSA mice are an invaluable tool to study mechanisms of GCI-associated neuro-degeneration. However, the specific full-blown pathology of MSA has been reproduced only by a double-hit approach combining transgenic GCIs and toxin-induced neuronal lesions [150], supporting the notion that exogenous environmental insults may be crucial to trigger MSA pathology in the presence of oligodendroglial α-synucleinopathy. Furthermore, the animal models have been important in studying novel therapeutic strategies for MSA.

Therapies

Principles of management

Currently, there is no effective neuroprotective therapy in MSA. Symptomatic treatment is restricted largely to parkinsonism and dysautonomia. Other features such as cerebellar ataxia appear to be unresponsive to drug treatment.

Neuroprotective therapy

A placebo-controlled double-blind pilot trial of recombinant human growth hormone (r-HGH) conducted by EMSA-SG has shown a trend toward reduction of motor progression (measured both with UPDRS and UMSARS) which, however, failed to reach significance [151].

More recently, minocycline, an antibiotic with neuroprotective effects in a transgenic MSA mouse model [152] as well as models of related neurodegenerative disorders [153,154], proved ineffective in a phase II neuroprotection trial by EMSA-SG and the German Parkinson Network (KNP) [9].

The primary and secondary endpoints of the randomized controlled double-blind NNIPPS (Neuroprotection and Natural History in Parkinson Plus Syndromes) trial investigating the effects of riluzole, an antiglutamatergic agent, on mortality and progression in AP including MSA have been negative [10]. A small randomized controlled trial had already excluded a symptomatic benefit of riluzole in a small series of MSA-P patients [155].

The success of further neuroprotection trials in MSA crucially depends on defining appropriate pathogenetic targets that are likely to mediate the progression of the disease [156]. Very recently, a multicenter neuroprotection trial with rasagiline, a MAO-B inhibitor, was launched in Europe and the United States.

Symptomatic therapy

Parkinsonism

Only a small number of randomized controlled trials have been conducted in MSA; the practical management is largely based on empirical evidence or single randomized studies.

Dopaminergic agents

L-dopa is widely regarded as the anti-parkinsonian therapy of choice in MSA although a randomized controlled trial of L-dopa has never been performed. Despite the fact that MSA patients are commonly believed to be non- or poorly responsive to dopaminergic therapy, efficacy often lasting for up to a few years has been documented in up to 40% of cases [1]. However, the benefit is transient in most of these subjects, leaving 90% of the MSA-P patients L-dopa unresponsive in the long term [26]. L-dopa responsiveness should be tested by administering escalating doses over a three-month period up to a least 1000 mg per day (if necessary and if tolerated) [6]. L-dopa-induced dyskinesias affecting orofacial and neck muscles occur in 50% of MSA-P patients, sometimes in the absence of motor benefit [157].

No randomized controlled trials with dopamine agonists are available; these compounds seem no more effective than L-dopa and are often poorly tolerated. Lisuride was effective in only one of seven MSA patients [158]. Heinz *et al.* reported the benefit of continuous subcutaneous lisuride infusion in four patients with OPCA and severe signs of parkinsonism [159]. Goetz and colleagues, using doses of 10–80 mg daily of bromocriptine, reported a benefit in five patients who had previously responded to L-dopa and in one patient who had failed to respond to L-dopa [160]. There are no reports on other ergolene or non-ergolene dopamine agonists such as pergolide, cabergoline, ropinirole, or pramipexole.

Pathological hypersexuality predominantly linked to adjuvant dopamine agonist therapy has been reported in two patients with MSA [161]. MSA patients frequently report the appearance or worsening of postural hypotension after initiation of dopaminergic therapy, which may limit further increase in dosage.

Anticholinergic agents

Anticholinergics usually do not improve motor symptoms, but they may be helpful when sialorrhea is severe and disturbing.

N-methyl D-aspartate receptor antagonists

Despite anecdotal benefit in single cases [14], a short-term open trial with amantadine at high doses (400–600 mg/day) in five patients with MSA unresponsive to L-dopa was negative [162]. These disappointing results were confirmed more recently in a randomized placebo-controlled trial [163].

Selective serotonin re-uptake inhibitors

Paroxetine 30 mg t.i.d. has been shown to improve motor symptoms in a randomized double-blind placebo-controlled trial with 19 MSA patients [164].

Surgical therapy

Whereas ablative neurosurgical procedures such as medial pallidotomy fail to improve parkinsonism in MSA [165], bilateral subthalamic stimulation has been reported beneficial in four patients with MSA-P [166] although a poor response was seen in other cases [167,168]. At present, there is no role for deep brain stimulation procedures in the routine management of MSA patients.

Non-pharmacological treatments

Because of the poor efficacy of anti-parkinsonian therapies in MSA, non-pharmacological interventions such as physical therapy, speech therapy, and occupational therapy are all the more important. Indeed, a recent study showed substantial benefit of occupational therapy in a series of 17 MSA patients [169]. Treated patients showed a reduction of 20% in UPDRS-ADL (activities of daily living) scores as well as the PDQ-39 index score whereas the control group deteriorated significantly over the two-month study period.

Dystonia

Local injections of botulinum toxin are effective in orofacial as well as limb dystonia associated with MSA [170]. Severe dysphagia with the necessity of nasogastric feeding has been reported after treatment of disproportionate antecollis with botulinum toxin, and this type of treatment is not recommended currently [171].

In addition, local botulinum toxin injections into the parotid and submandibular glands have been effective in PD-associated sialorrhea in two double-blind placebo-controlled trials [172,173]. In contrast to anticholinergics, central side-effects can be avoided.

Autonomic symptoms

Treatment of autonomic dysfunction is crucial to avoid complications like ascending urinary tract infections or OH, which could lead to falls. In addition, autonomic dysfunction is associated with reduced quality of life [27,174]. Unfortunately, most of the available therapies have not been evaluated in randomized controlled trials.

Orthostatic hypotension

Non-pharmacological options to treat OH include sufficient fluid intake, high-salt diet, more frequent but smaller meals per day to reduce postprandial hypotension by spreading the total carbohydrate intake, and compression stockings or custom-made elastic body garments. Ingestion of approx. 0.5 L of water in less than five minutes substantially raises blood pressure in patients with autonomic failure including MSA [175,176]. During the night, head-up tilt not only reduces hypertensive cerebral perfusion pressure but also increases intravasal volume up to 1 L within a week, which is particularly helpful in improving hypotension early in the morning. Constipation can affect overall well-being and is relieved by an increase in intraluminal fluid, which may be achieved by macrogol-water solution [177].

Midodrine showed significant benefit in randomized placebo-controlled trials [178,179] in patients with OH but may exacerbate urinary retention. Another promising drug seems to be the noradrenaline precursor l-threodihydroxy-phenylserine (l-threo-DOPS), which has been used for this indication in Japan for years and the efficacy of which has now been shown by two double-blind placebo-controlled trials including patients with MSA [180,181].

The somatostatin analogue, octreotide, has been shown to be beneficial in postprandial hypotension in patients with pure autonomical failure [182], presumably because it inhibits the release of vasodilatory gastrointestinal peptides [183]; importantly, it does not enhance nocturnal hypertension [182].

Urinary dysfunction

Whereas procholinergic substances are usually not successful in adequately reducing postvoid residual volume in MSA, anticholinergic drugs like oxybutynin can improve symptoms of detrusor hyperreflexia or sphincter–detrusor dyssynergy in the early course of the disease [30]. However, central side-effects may be limiting. In a large multicenter randomized controlled study in patients with detrusor hyperreflexia, trospium chloride, a peripherally acting quaternary anticholinergic, has been shown to be equally effective with better tolerability [184]. However, trospium has not been investigated in MSA and, furthermore, it appears that central and peripheral anticholinergics are equally effective and tolerated in non-demented PD patients. At present, there is no evidence for ranking the efficacy and safety of anticholinergic drugs in the management of detrusor hyperreflexia associated with MSA. Alpha-adrenergic receptor antagonists like prazosin and moxisylyte have been shown to improve voiding with reduction of residual volumes in MSA patients [185].

The vasopressin analogue desmopressin, which acts on renal tubular vasopressin-2 receptors, reduces nocturnal polyuria and improves morning postural hypotension [186].

The peptide erythropoietin may be beneficial in some patients by raising red blood cell mass, secondarily improving cerebral oxygenation [187,188].

Surgical therapies for neurogenic bladder problems should be avoided in MSA, because postoperatively worsening bladder control is most likely [30], but severe prostate hypertrophy with urinary retention and secondary hydronephrosis, for example, cannot be left untreated.

With postmicturition volumes greater than 150 mL, clean intermittent catheterization three to four times per day may be necessary to prevent secondary consequences. A permanent transcutaneous suprapubic catheter may become necessary if mechanical obstruction in the urethra or motor symptoms of MSA prevent uncomplicated catheterization.

Erectile dysfunction

After an initial report on the efficacy of the treatment of erectile dysfunction in PD [189], sildenafil citrate has been shown to be effective in a randomized double-blind placebo-controlled trial in patients with PD and MSA [190]. Because it may unmask or exacerbate OH, measurement of lying and standing blood pressure before prescribing sildenafil to men with parkinsonism is recommended. Erectile failure in MSA may also be improved by oral yohimbine, intracavernosal injection of papaverine, or a penis implant [30].

Inspiratory stridor

Inspiratory stridor develops in about 30% of patients. Continuous positive airway pressure (CPAP) may be helpful in some of these patients, and suitable as long-term therapy [191–193]. A tracheostomy is rarely needed or performed.

Palliative care

Because the results of drug treatment for MSA are generally poor, other therapies are all the more important. Physical therapy helps maintain mobility and prevent contractures, and speech therapy can improve speech and swallowing, and provide communication aids [169]. Dysphagia may require feeding by means of a nasogastric tube or even percutaneous endoscopic gastrostomy. Occupational therapy helps to limit the handicap resulting from the patient's disabilities and should include a home visit. Provision of a wheelchair is usually dictated by the liability to falls because of postural instability and gait ataxia but not by akinesia and rigidity per se. Psychological support for patients and partners needs to be stressed.

Pragmatic management

Parkinsonism

    1st choice: L-dopa (up to 1000 mg/day, if tolerated and necessary)
    2nd choice: dopamine agonists (PD titration schemes)
    3rd choice: amantadine: (100 mg t.i.d.)

Dystonia (orofacial and limb, antecollis excluded)

    1st choice: botulinum toxin

Cerebellar ataxia

    None available

Autonomic symptoms

Orthostatic hypotension

1st choice: nonpharmacological strategies, e.g. elastic support stockings or tights, high-salt diet, frequent small meals, head-up tilt of the bed at night

If needed: add fludrocortisone (0.1–0.3 mg) at night

If needed: add midodrine (2.5–10 mg t.i.d.) (combined with fludrocortisone)

If needed: replace midodrine by ephedrine (15–45 mg t.i.d.) or L-threo-DOPS (100 mg t.i.d.)

Urinary failure – urge incontinence

Trospium chloride (20 mg b.i.d. or 15 mg t.i.d.)

Oxybutynin (2.5–5 mg b.i.d. to t.i.d.). NB central side-effects

Urinary failure – incomplete bladder emptying

Postmicturition residue of >100 mL is an indication for intermittent self-catheterization

In the advanced stages of MSA, a urethral or suprapubic catheter may become necessary

Erectile failure

1st choice: sildenafil (50–100 mg)

2nd choice: oral yohimbine (2.5–5 mg)

3rd choice: intracavernosal injection of papaverine

Palliative therapy

- Physical therapy
- Occupational therapy
- Speech therapy
- Percutaneous endoscopic gastrostomy (PEG)
- Botulinum toxin for sialorrhea
- CPAP (for prominent stridor)
- Tracheostomy (rarely needed)

References

1. Wenning GK, Colosimo C, Geser F, et al. Multiple system atrophy. *Lancet Neurol* 2004; **3**(2): 93–103.
2. Graham JG, Oppenheimer DR. Orthostatic hypotension and nicotine sensitivity in a case of multiple system atrophy. *J Neurol Neurosurg Psychiatry* 1969; **32**(1): 28–34.
3. Papp MI, Kahn JE, Lantos PL. Glial cytoplasmic inclusions in the CNS of patients with multiple system atrophy (striatonigral degeneration, olivopontocerebellar atrophy and Shy-Drager syndrome). *J Neurol Sci* 1989; **94**(1–3): 79–100.
4. Quinn N. Multiple system atrophy the nature of the beast. *J Neurol Neurosurg Psychiatry* 1989; Suppl: 78–89.
5. Gilman S, Low P, Quinn N, et al. Consensus statement on the diagnosis of multiple system atrophy. *Clin Auton Res* 1998; **8**: 359–62.
6. Gilman S, Wenning GK, Low PA, et al. Second consensus statement on the diagnosis of multiple system atrophy. *Neurology* 2008; **71**(9): 670–6.
7. Wenning GK, Tison F, Seppi K, et al. Development and validation of the Unified Multiple System Atrophy Rating Scale (UMSARS). *Mov Disord* 2004; **19**(12): 1391–402.

8. Stefanova N, Tison F, Reindl M, et al. Animal models of multiple system atrophy. *Trends Neurosci* 2005; **28**(9): 501–6.

9. Dodel R, Spottke A, Gerhard A, et al. Minocycline 1 Year Therapy in Multiple-System-Atrophy: Effect on Clinical Symptoms and [11C] (R)-PK11195 PET (MEMSA-Trial). *Mov Disord* 2010; 25(1): 97–107.

10. Aarsland D, Anderson K, Larsen JP, et al. Prevalence and characteristics of dementia in Parkinson disease: an 8-year prospective study. *Arch Neurol* 2003; **60**(3): 387–92.

11. Gilman S, May SJ, Shults CW, et al. The North American Multiple System Atrophy Study Group. *J Neural Transm* 2005; **112**: 1687–94.

12. Scholz SW, Houlden H, Schulte C, et al. SNCA variants are associated with increased risk for multiple system atrophy. *Ann Neurol* 2009; **65**(5): 610–14.

13. Hara K, Momose Y, Tokiguchi S, et al. Multiplex families with multiple system atrophy. *Arch Neurol* 2007; **64**: 545–51.

14. Wenning GK, Ben Shlomo Y, Magalhaes M, et al. Clinical features and natural history of multiple system atrophy. An analysis of 100 cases. *Brain* 1994; **117** (4): 835–45.

15. Bower JH, Maraganore DM, McDonnell SK, et al. Incidence of progressive supranuclear palsy and multiple system atrophy in Olmsted County, Minnesota, 1976 to 1990. *Neurology* 1997; **49**(5): 1284–8.

16. Schrag A, Ben-Shlomo Y, Quinn NP. Prevalence of progressive supranuclear palsy and multiple system atrophy: a cross-sectional study. *Lancet* 1999; **354**: 1771–5.

17. Köllensperger M, Geser F, Ndayisaba JP, et al. Clinical presentation, diagnosis and management of MSA in Europe: data from the EMSA-SG registry. *Mov Disord* 2010 [E pub ahead of print].

18. Watanabe H, Saito Y, Terao S, et al. Progression and prognosis in multiple system atrophy: an analysis of 230 Japanese patients. *Brain* 2002; **125**: 1070–83.

19. Tsuji S, Onodera O, Goto J, et al. Sporadic ataxias in Japan – a population-based epidemiological study. *Cerebellum* 2008; 7(2): 189–97.

20. Sakakibara R, Hattori T, Uchiyama T, et al. Urinary dysfunction and orthostatic hypotension in multiple system atrophy: which is the more common and earlier manifestation? *J Neurol Neurosurg Psychiatry* 2000; **68**(1): 65–9.

21. Trojanowski JQ, Revesz T. Proposed neuropathological criteria for the post mortem diagnosis of multiple system atrophy. *Neuropathol Appl Neurobiol* 2007; **33**(6): 615–20.

22. Schrag A, Wenning GK, Quinn N, et al. Survival in multiple system atrophy. *Mov Disord* 2008; **23**(2): 294–6.

23. O'Sullivan SS, Massey LA, Williams DR, et al. Clinical outcomes of progressive supranuclear palsy and multiple system atrophy. *Brain* 2008; **131**(5): 1362–72.

24. Ben Shlomo Y, Wenning GK, Tison F, et al. Survival of patients with pathologically proven multiple system atrophy: a meta-analysis. *Neurology* 1997; **48**: 384–93.

25. Tada M, Kakita A, Toyoshima Y, et al. Depletion of medullary serotonergic neurons in patients with multiple system atrophy who succumbed to sudden death. *Brain* 2009; **132**: 1810–19.

26. Geser F, Wenning GK, Seppi K, et al. Progression of multiple system atrophy (MSA): a prospective natural history study by the European MSA Study Group (EMSA SG). *Mov Disord* 2006; **21**(2): 179–86.

27. Kollensperger M, Stampfer-Kountchev M, Seppi K, et al. Progression of dysautonomia in multiple system atrophy: a prospective study of self-perceived impairment. *Eur J Neurol* 2007; **14**(1): 66–72.

28. Gibbons CH, Freeman R. Delayed orthostatic hypotension: a frequent cause of orthostatic intolerance. *Neurology* 2006; **67**: 28–32.

29. Lipp A, Sandroni P, Ahlskog JE, et al. Prospective differentiation of multiple system atrophy from Parkinson disease, with and without autonomic failure. *Arch Neurol* 2009; **66**: 742–50.

30. Beck RO, Betts CD, Fowler CJ. Genitourinary dysfunction in multiple system atrophy: clinical features and treatment in 62 cases. *J Urol* 1994; **151**: 1336–41.

31. Sakakibara R, Hattori T, Uchiyama T, et al. Videourodynamic and sphincter motor unit potential analyses in Parkinson's disease and multiple system atrophy. *J Neurol Neurosurg Psychiatry* 2001; **71**: 600–6.

32. Vodusek DB. How to diagnose MSA early: the role of sphincter EMG. *J Neural Transm* 2005; **112**: 1657–68.

33. Sakakibara R, Uchiyama T, Yamanishi T, et al. Sphincter EMG as a diagnostic tool in autonomic disorders. *Clin Auton Res* 2009; **19**: 20–31.

34. Abdo WF, van de Warrenburg BP, Munneke M, et al. CSF analysis differentiates multiple-system atrophy from idiopathic late-onset cerebellar ataxia. *Neurology* 2006; **67**: 474–9.

35. Brettschneider J, Petzold A, Süssmuth SD, et al. Neurofilament heavy-chain NfH(SMI35) in cerebrospinal fluid supports the differential diagnosis of Parkinsonian syndromes. *Mov Disord* 2006; **21**: 2224–7.

36. Abdo WF, Bloem BR, Van Geel WJ, et al. CSF neurofilament light chain and tau differentiate multiple system atrophy from Parkinson's disease. *Neurobiol Aging* 2007; **28**: 742–7.

37. Petzold A, Thompson EJ, Keir G, et al. Longitudinal one-year study of levels and stoichiometry of neurofilament heavy and light chain concentrations in CSF in patients with multiple system atrophy. *J Neurol Sci* 2009; **279**: 76–9.

38. Kimber JR, Watson L, Mathias CJ. Distinction of idiopathic Parkinson's disease from multiple-system atrophy by stimulation of growth-hormone release with clonidine. *Lancet* 1997; **349**: 1877–81.

39. Pellecchia MT, Longo K, Pivonello R, et al. Multiple system atrophy is distinguished from idiopathic Parkinson's disease by the arginine growth hormone stimulation test. *Ann Neurol* 2006; **60**(5): 611–15.

40. Pellecchia MT, Pivonello R, Colao A, et al. Growth hormone stimulation tests in the differential diagnosis of Parkinson's disease. *Clin Med Res* 2006; **4**(4): 322–5.

41. Brooks DJ, Seppi K. Proposed neuroimaging criteria for the diagnosis of multiple system atrophy. *Mov Disord* 2009; **24**(7): 949–64.

42. Walter U, Niehaus L, Probst T, et al. Brain parenchyma sonography discriminates Parkinson's disease and atypical parkinsonian syndromes. *Neurology* 2003; **60**: 74–7.

43. Walter U, Dressler D, Probst T, et al. Transcranial brain sonography findings in discriminating between parkinsonism and idiopathic Parkinson disease. *Arch Neurol* 2007; **64**: 1635–40.

44. Schrag A, Good CD, Miszkiel K, et al. Differentiation of atypical parkinsonian syndromes with routine MRI. *Neurology* 2000; **54**: 697–702.

45. Quattrone A, Nicoletti G, Messina D, et al. MR imaging index for differentiation of progressive supranuclear palsy from Parkinson disease and the Parkinson variant of multiple system atrophy. *Radiology* 2008; **246**: 214–21.

46. Paviour DC, Price SL, Jahanshahi M, et al. Regional brain volumes distinguish PSP, MSA-P, and PD: MRI-based clinico-radiological correlations. *Mov Disord* 2006; **21**(7): 989–96.

47. Paviour DC, Price SL, Jahanshahi M, et al. Longitudinal MRI in progressive supranuclear palsy and multiple system atrophy: rates and regions of atrophy. *Brain* 2006; **129**(4): 1040–9.

48. Brenneis C, Egger K, Scherfler C, et al. Progression of brain atrophy in multiple system atrophy. A longitudinal VBM study. *J Neurol* 2007; **254**(2): 191–6.

49. Schocke MF, Seppi K, Esterhammer R, et al. Diffusion-weighted MRI differentiates the Parkinson variant of multiple system atrophy from PD. *Neurology* 2002; **58**: 575–80.

50. Seppi K, Schocke MF, Esterhammer R, et al. Diffusion-weighted imaging discriminates progressive supranuclear palsy from PD, but not from the Parkinson variant of multiple system atrophy. *Neurology* 2003; **60**(6): 922–7.

51. Nicoletti G, Lodi R, Condino F, et al. Apparent diffusion coefficient measurements of the middle cerebellar peduncle differentiate the Parkinson variant of MSA from Parkinson's disease and progressive supranuclear palsy. *Brain* 2006; **129**(10): 2679–87.

52. Paviour DC, Thornton JS, Lees AJ, et al. Diffusion-weighted magnetic resonance imaging differentiates Parkinsonian variant of multiple-system atrophy from progressive supranuclear palsy. *Mov Disord* 2007; **22**(1): 68–74.

53. Gilman S. Functional imaging with positron emission tomography in multiple

system atrophy. *J Neural Transm* 2005; **112**(12): 1647–55.

54. Scherfler C, Seppi K, Donnemiller E, et al. Voxel-wise analysis of [123I]beta-CIT SPECT differentiates the Parkinson variant of multiple system atrophy from idiopathic Parkinson's disease. *Brain* 2005; **128**: 1605–12.

55. Gerhard A, Banati RB, Goerres GB, et al. [11C](R)-PK11195 PET imaging of microglial activation in multiple system atrophy. *Neurology* 2003; **61**(5): 686–9.

56. Eidelberg D, Takikawa S, Moeller JR, et al. Striatal hypometabolism distinguishes striatonigral degeneration from Parkinson's disease. *Ann Neurol* 1993; **33**(5): 518–27.

57. Gilman S, Koeppe RA, Junck L, et al. Patterns of cerebral glucose metabolism detected with positron emission tomography differ in multiple system atrophy and olivopontocerebellar atrophy. *Ann Neurol* 1994; **36**(2): 166–75.

58. Perani D, Bressi S, Testa D, et al. Clinical/metabolic correlations in multiple system atrophy. A fludeoxyglucose F 18 positron emission tomographic study. *Arch Neurol* 1995; **52**(2): 179–85.

59. Eckert T, Tang C, Ma Y, et al. Abnormal metabolic networks in atypical parkinsonism. *Mov Disord* 2008; **23**: 727–33.

60. Kwon KY, Choi CG, Kim JS, et al. Comparison of brain MRI and 18F-FDG PET in the differential diagnosis of multiple system atrophy from Parkinson's disease. *Mov Disord* 2007; **22**(16): 2352–8.

61. Braune S, Reinhardt M, Schnitzer R, et al. Cardiac uptake of [123I]MIBG separates Parkinson's disease from multiple system atrophy. *Neurology* 1999; **53**: 1020–5.

62. Braune S. The role of cardiac metaiodobenzylguanidine uptake in the differential diagnosis of parkinsonian syndromes. *Clin Auton Res* 2001; **11**: 351–5.

63. Courbon F, Brefel-Courbon C, Thalamas C, et al. Cardiac MIBG scintigraphy is a sensitive tool for detecting cardiac sympathetic denervation in Parkinson's disease. *Mov Disord* 2003; **18**(8): 890–7.

64. Goldstein DS, Holmes C, Cannon RO 3rd, et al. Sympathetic cardioneuropathy in dysautonomias. *N Engl J Med* 1997; **336**(10): 696–702.

65. Kollensperger M, Seppi K, Liener C, et al. Diffusion weighted imaging best discriminates PD from MSA-P: A comparison with tilt table testing and heart MIBG scintigraphy. *Mov Disord* 2007; **22**(12): 1771–6.

66. Orimo S, Kanazawa T, Nakamura A, et al. Degeneration of cardiac sympathetic nerve can occur in multiple system atrophy. *Acta Neuropathol* 2007; **113**: 81–6.

67. Daniel S. The neuropathology and neurochemistry of multiple system atrophy. In: Mathias CJ, Bartko JJ, eds. *Autonomic failure*. Oxford: Oxford University Press, 1999; 321–8.

68. Jellinger KA. Neuropathological spectrum of synucleinopathies. *Mov Disord* 2003; **18**(Suppl 6): S2–12.

69. Kume A, Takahashi A, Hashizume Y, et al. Neuronal cell loss of the striatonigral system in multiple system atrophy. *J Neurol Sci* 1993; **117**: 33–40.

70. Wenning GK, Tison F, Ben Shlomo Y, et al. Multiple system atrophy: a review of 203 pathologically proven cases. *Mov Disord* 1997; **12**: 133–47.

71. Berciano J, Monton FI, Maeso MC, et al. [Man aged 49 years suffering from progressive clinical picture with palatal tremor, segmental myoclonus, ataxia, parkinsonism, amyotrophy, pyramidal signs, supranuclear ophthalmoplegia and cognitive decline]. *Neurologia* 2002; **17**: 237–43.

72. Jellinger KA, Seppi K, Wenning GK. Grading of neuropathology in multiple system atrophy: proposal for a novel scale. *Mov Disord* 2005; **20**(Suppl 12): S29–36.

73. Wakabayashi K, Mori F, Nishie M, et al. An autopsy case of early ("minimal change") olivopontocerebellar atrophy (multiple system atrophy-cerebellar). *Acta Neuropathol* 2005; **110**: 185–90.

74. Benarroch EE, Schmeichel AM, Sandroni P. et al. Involvement of vagal autonomic nuclei in multiple system atrophy and Lewy body disease. *Neurology* 2006; **66**: 378–83.

75. Benarroch EE. Brainstem in multiple system atrophy: clinicopathological correlations. *Cell Mol Neurobiol* 2003; **23**: 519–26.

76. Benarroch EE, Schmeichel AM, Low PA, et al. Involvement of medullary

serotonergic groups in multiple system atrophy. *Ann Neurol* 2004; **55**: 418–22.

77. Papp MI, Lantos PL. The distribution of oligodendroglial inclusions in multiple system atrophy and its relevance to clinical symptomatology. *Brain* 1994; **117** (2): 235–43.

78. Schmeichel AM, Buchhalter LC, Low PA, et al. Mesopontine cholinergic neuron involvement in Lewy body dementia and multiple system atrophy. *Neurology* 2008; **70**: 368–73.

79. Shy GM, Drager GA. A neurological syndrome associated with orthostatic hypotension: a clinical-pathologic study. *Arch Neurol* 1960; **2**: 511–27.

80. Benarroch EE, Schmeichel AM, Sandroni P, et al. Involvement of hypocretin neurons in multiple system atrophy. *Acta Neuropathol* 2007; **113**: 75–80.

81. Nishie M, Mori F, Yoshimoto M, et al. A quantitative investigation of neuronal cytoplasmic and intranuclear inclusions in the pontine and inferior olivary nuclei in multiple system atrophy. *Neuropathol Appl Neurobiol* 2004; **30**: 546–54.

82. Sone M, Yoshida M, Hashizume Y, et al. alpha-Synuclein-immunoreactive structure formation is enhanced in sympathetic ganglia of patients with multiple system atrophy. *Acta Neuropathol* (Berl) 2005; **110**: 19–26.

83. Konno H, Yamamoto T, Iwasaki Y, et al. Shy-Drager syndrome and amyotrophic lateral sclerosis. Cytoarchitectonic and morphometric studies of sacral autonomic neurons. *J Neurol Sci* 1986; **73**: 193–204.

84. Ozawa T. Morphological substrate of autonomic failure and neurohormonal dysfunction in multiple system atrophy: impact on determining phenotype spectrum. *Acta Neuropathol* 2007; **114**: 201–11.

85. Yamamoto T, Sakakibara R, Uchiyama T, et al. When is Onuf's nucleus involved in multiple system atrophy? A sphincter electromyography study. *J Neurol Neurosurg Psychiatry* 2005; **76**: 1645–8.

86. Lantos PL. The definition of multiple system atrophy: a review of recent developments. *J Neuropathol Exp Neurol* 1998; **57**: 1099–111.

87. Spillantini MG, Crowther RA, Jakes R, et al. Filamentous alpha-synuclein inclusions link multiple system atrophy with Parkinson's disease and dementia with Lewy bodies. *Neurosci Lett* 1998; **251**: 205–8.

88. Tu PH, Galvin JE, Baba M, et al. Glial cytoplasmic inclusions in white matter oligodendrocytes of multiple system atrophy brains contain insoluble alpha-synuclein. *Ann Neurol* 1998; **44**: 415–22.

89. Wakabayashi K, Yoshimoto M, Tsuji S, et al. Alpha-synuclein immunoreactivity in glial cytoplasmic inclusions in multiple system atrophy. *Neurosci Lett* 1998; **249**: 180–2.

90. Dickson DW, Lin W, Liu WK, et al. Multiple system atrophy: a sporadic synucleinopathy. *Brain Pathol* 1999; **9**: 721–32.

91. Inoue M, Yagishita S, Ryo M, et al. The distribution and dynamic density of oligodendroglial cytoplasmic inclusions (GCIs) in multiple system atrophy: a correlation between the density of GCIs and the degree of involvement of striatonigral and olivopontocerebellar systems. *Acta Neuropathol* (Berl) 1997; **93**: 585–91.

92. Ozawa T, Paviour D, Quinn NP, et al. The spectrum of pathological involvement of the striatonigral and olivopontocerebellar systems in multiple system atrophy: clinicopathological correlations. *Brain* 2004; **127**: 2657–71.

93. Arima K, Murayama S, Mukoyama M, et al. Immunocytochemical and ultrastructural studies of neuronal and oligodendroglial cytoplasmic inclusions in multiple system atrophy. 1. Neuronal cytoplasmic inclusions. *Acta Neuropathol* 1992; **83**: 453–60.

94. Armstrong RA, Cairns NJ, Lantos PL. Multiple system atrophy (MSA): topographic distribution of the alpha-synuclein-associated pathological changes. *Parkinsonism Relat Disord* 2006; **12**: 356–62.

95. Armstrong RA, Lantos PL, Cairns NJ. Spatial patterns of alpha-synuclein positive glial cytoplasmic inclusions in multiple system atrophy. *Mov Disord* 2004; **19**: 109–12.

96. Kato S, Nakamura H. Cytoplasmic argyrophilic inclusions in neurons of pontine nuclei in patients

with olivopontocerebellar atrophy: immunohistochemical and ultrastructural studies. *Acta Neuropathol* 1990; **79**: 584–94.

97. Papp MI, Lantos PL. Accumulation of tubular structures in oligodendroglial and neuronal cells as the basic alteration in multiple system atrophy. *J Neurol Sci* 1992; **107**: 172–82.

98. Sakurai A, Okamoto K, Yaguchi M, et al. Pathology of the inferior olivary nucleus in patients with multiple system atrophy. *Acta Neuropathol* (Berl) 2002; **103**: 550–4.

99. Takeda A, Arai N, Komori T, et al. Tau immunoreactivity in glial cytoplasmic inclusions in multiple system atrophy. *Neurosci Lett* 1997; **234**: 63–6.

100. Yokoyama T, Kusunoki JI, Hasegawa K, et al. Distribution and dynamic process of neuronal cytoplasmic inclusion (NCI) in MSA: correlation of the density of NCI and the degree of involvement of the pontine nuclei. *Neuropathology* 2001; **21**: 145–54.

101. Wenning GK, Stefanova N, Jellinger KA, et al. Multiple system atrophy: a primary oligodendrogliopathy. *Ann Neurol* 2008; **64**: 239–46.

102. Solano SM, Miller DW, Augood SJ, et al. Expression of alpha-synuclein, parkin, and ubiquitin carboxy-terminal hydrolase L1 mRNA in human brain: genes associated with familial Parkinson's disease. *Ann Neurol* 2000; **47**: 201–10.

103. Kahle PJ, Neumann M, Ozmen L, et al. Hyperphosphorylation and insolubility of alpha-synuclein in transgenic mouse oligodendrocytes. *EMBO Rep* 2002; **3**: 583–8.

104. Shults CW, Rockenstein E, Crews L, et al. Neurological and neurodegenerative alterations in a transgenic mouse model expressing human alpha-synuclein under oligodendrocyte promoter: implications for multiple system atrophy. *J Neurosci* 2005; **25**: 10689–99.

105. Yazawa I, Giasson BI, Sasaki R, et al. Mouse model of multiple system atrophy alpha-synuclein expression in oligodendrocytes causes glial and neuronal degeneration. *Neuron* 2005; **45**: 847–59.

106. Miller DW, Johnson JM, Solano SM, et al. Absence of alpha-synuclein mRNA expression in normal and multiple system atrophy oligodendroglia. *J Neural Transm* 2005; **112**: 1613–24.

107. Jellinger KA. p25alpha immunoreactivity in multiple system atrophy and Parkinson disease. *Acta Neuropathol* 2006; **112**: 112.

108. Kovacs GG, Gelpi E, Lehotzky A, et al. The brain-specific protein TPPP/ p25 in pathological protein deposits of neurodegenerative diseases. *Acta Neuropathol* 2007; **113**: 153–61.

109. Lindersson E, Lundvig D, Petersen C, et al. p25alpha Stimulates alpha-synuclein aggregation and is co-localized with aggregated alpha-synuclein in alpha-synucleinopathies. *J Biol Chem* 2005 **280**: 5703–15.

110. Song YJ, Lundvig DM, Huang Y, et al. p25alpha relocalizes in oligodendroglia from myelin to cytoplasmic inclusions in multiple system atrophy. *Am J Pathol* 2007; **171**: 1291–303.

111. Matsuo A, Akiguchi I, Lee GC, et al. Myelin degeneration in multiple system atrophy detected by unique antibodies. *Am J Pathol* 1998; **153**: 735–44.

112. Probst-Cousin S, Rickert CH, Schmid KW, et al. Cell death mechanisms in multiple system atrophy. *J Neuropathol Exp Neurol* 1998; **57**: 814–21.

113. Wakabayashi K, Takahashi H. Cellular pathology in multiple system atrophy. *Neuropathology* 2006; **26**: 338–45.

114. Yoshida M. Multiple system atrophy: alpha-synuclein and neuronal degeneration. *Neuropathology* 2007; **27**: 484–93.

115. Ishizawa K, Komori T, Sasaki S, et al. Microglial activation parallels system degeneration in multiple system atrophy. *J Neuropathol Exp Neurol* 2004; **63**: 43–52.

116. Schwarz J, Weis S, Kraft E, et al. Signal changes on MRI and increases in reactive microgliosis, astrogliosis, and iron in the putamen of two patients with multiple system atrophy. *J Neurol Neurosurg Psychiatry* 1996; **60**: 98–101.

117. Brown RC, Lockwood AH, Sonawane BR. Neurodegenerative diseases: an overview of environmental risk factors. *Environ Health Perspect* 2005; **113**: 1250–6.

118. Hanna PA, Jankovic J, Kirkpatrick JB. Multiple system atrophy: the putative

causative role of environmental toxins. *Arch Neurol* 1999; **56**: 90–4.

119. Nee LE, Gomez MR, Dambrosia J, et al. Environmental-occupational risk factors and familial associations in multiple system atrophy: a preliminary investigation. *Clin Auton Res* 1991; **1**: 9–13.

120. Vanacore N. Epidemiological evidence on multiple system atrophy. *J Neural Transm* 2005; **112**: 1605–12.

121. Chrysostome V, Tison F, Yekhlef F, et al. Epidemiology of multiple system atrophy: a prevalence and pilot risk factor study in Aquitaine, France. *Neuroepidemiology* 2004; **23**: 201–8.

122. Vidal JS, Vidailhet M, Elbaz A, et al. Risk factors of multiple system atrophy: a case-control study in French patients. *Mov Disord* 2008; **23**: 797–803.

123. Galanaud JP, Elbaz A, Clavel J, et al. Cigarette smoking and Parkinson's disease: a case-control study in a population characterized by a high prevalence of pesticide exposure. *Mov Disord* 2005; **20**: 181–9.

124. Vanacore N, Bonifati V, Fabbrini G, et al. Smoking habits in multiple system atrophy and progressive supranuclear palsy. European Study Group on Atypical Parkinsonisms. *Neurology* 2000; **54**: 114–19.

125. Wenning GK, Wagner S, Daniel S, et al. Multiple system atrophy: sporadic or familial? *Lancet* 1993; **342**: 681.

126. Soma H, Yabe I, Takei A, et al. Heredity in multiple system atrophy. *J Neurol Sci* 2006; **240**: 107–10.

127. Wullner U, Abele M, Schmitz-Huebsch T, et al. Probable multiple system atrophy in a German family. *J Neurol Neurosurg Psychiatry* 2004; **75**: 924–5.

128. Gilman S, Sima AA, Junck L, et al. Spinocerebellar ataxia type 1 with multiple system degeneration and glial cytoplasmic inclusions. *Ann Neurol* 1996; **39**: 241–55.

129. Kamm C, Healy DG, Quinn NP, et al. The fragile X tremor ataxia syndrome in the differential diagnosis of multiple system atrophy: data from the EMSA Study Group. *Brain* 2005; **128**: 1855–60.

130. Khan NL, Giunti P, Sweeney MG, et al. Parkinsonism and nigrostriatal dysfunction are associated with

spinocerebellar ataxia type 6 (SCA6). *Mov Disord* 2005; **20**: 1115–19.

131. Lee WY, Jin DK, Oh MR, et al. Frequency analysis and clinical characterization of spinocerebellar ataxia types 1, 2, 3, 6, and 7 in Korean patients. *Arch Neurol* 2003; **60**: 858–63.

132. Nirenberg MJ, Libien J, Vonsattel JP, et al. Multiple system atrophy in a patient with the spinocerebellar ataxia 3 gene mutation. *Mov Disord* 2007; **22**: 251–4.

133. Lincoln SJ, Ross OA, Milkovic NM, et al. Quantitative PCR-based screening of alpha-synuclein multiplication in multiple system atrophy. *Parkinsonism Relat Disord* 2007; **13**: 340–2.

134. Morris HR, Vaughan JR, Datta SR, et al. Multiple system atrophy/progressive supranuclear palsy: alpha-Synuclein, synphilin, tau, and APOE. *Neurology* 2000; **55**: 1918–20.

135. Ozawa T. Pathology and genetics of multiple system atrophy: an approach to determining genetic susceptibility spectrum. *Acta Neuropathol* (Berl) 2006; **112**: 531–8.

136. Ozawa T, Takano H, Onodera O, et al. No mutation in the entire coding region of the alpha-synuclein gene in pathologically confirmed cases of multiple system atrophy. *Neurosci Lett* 1999; **270**: 110–12.

137. Al-Chalabi A, Dürr A, Wood NW, et al. NNIPPS Genetic Study Group. Genetic variants of the alpha-synuclein gene SNCA are associated with multiple system atrophy. *PLoS One* 2009; **4**(9): e7114.

138. Scholz SW, Houlden H, Sculte C, et al. SNCA variants are associated with increased risk of multiple system atrophy. *Ann Neurol* 2009; **65**(5): 610–14.

139. Combarros O, Infante J, Llorca, et al. Interleukin-1A (-889) genetic polymorphism increases the risk of multiple system atrophy. *Mov Disord* 2003; **18**: 1385–6.

140. Furiya Y, Hirano M, Kurumatani N, et al. Alpha-1-antichymotrypsin gene polymorphism and susceptibility to multiple system atrophy (MSA). *Brain Res Mol Brain Res* 2005; **138**: 178–81.

141. Infante J, Llorca J, Berciano J, et al. Interleukin-8, intercellular adhesion molecule-1 and tumour necrosis

factor-alpha gene polymorphisms and the risk for multiple system atrophy. *J Neurol Sci* 2005; **228**: 11–13.

142. Nishimura M, Kawakami H, Komure O, et al. Contribution of the interleukin-1beta gene polymorphism in multiple system atrophy. *Mov Disord* 2002; **17**: 808–11.

143. Nishimura M, Kuno S, Kaji R, et al. Influence of a tumor necrosis factor gene polymorphism in Japanese patients with multiple system atrophy. *Neurosci Lett* 2005; **374**: 218–21.

144. Soma H, Yabe I, Takei A, et al. Associations between multiple system atrophy and polymorphisms of SLC1A4, SQSTM1, and EIF4EBP1 genes. *Mov Disord* 2008; **23**: 1161–7.

145. Fernagut PO, Diguet E, Stefanova N, et al. Subacute systemic 3-nitropropionic acid intoxication induces a distinct motor disorder in adult C57B1/6 mice: Behavioural and histopathological characterisation. *Neuroscience* 2002; **114**: 1005–17.

146. Scherfler C, Puschban Z, Ghorayeb I, et al. Complex motor disturbances in a sequential double lesion rat model of striatonigral degeneration (multiple system atrophy). *Neuroscience* 2000; **99**: 43–54.

147. Stefanova N, Lundblad M, Tison F, et al. Effects of pulsatile L-DOPA treatment in the double lesion rat model of striatonigral degeneration (multiple system atrophy). *Neurobiol Dis* 2004; **15**: 630–9.

148. Stefanova N, Puschban Z, Fernagut PO, et al. Neuropathological and behavioral changes induced by various treatment paradigms with MPTP and 3-nitropropionic acid in mice: towards a model of striatonigral degeneration (multiple system atrophy). *Acta Neuropathol* (Berl) 2003; **106**: 157–66.

149. Wenning GK, Granata R, Laboyrie PM, et al. Reversal of behavioural abnormalities by fetal allografts in a novel rat model of striatonigral degeneration. *Mov Disord* 1996; **11**: 522–32.

150. Stefanova N, Reindl M, Neumann M, et al. Oxidative stress in transgenic mice with oligodendroglial alpha-synuclein overexpression replicates the characteristic neuropathology of multiple system atrophy. *Am J Pathol* 2005; **166**: 869–76.

151. Holmberg B, Johansson JO, Poewe W, et al. Safety and tolerability of growth hormone therapy in multiple system atrophy: a double-blind, placebo-controlled study. *Mov Disord* 2007; **22**(8): 1138–44.

152. Stefanova N, Reindl M, Neumann M, et al. Microglial activation mediates neurodegeneration related to oligodendroglial alpha-synucleinopathy: implications for multiple system atrophy. *Mov Disord* 2007; **22**(15): 2196–203.

153. Zhu S, Stavrovskaya IG, Drozda M, et al. Minocycline inhibits cytochrome c release and delays progression of amyotrophic lateral sclerosis in mice. *Nature* 2002; **417**: 74–8.

154. Casarejos MJ, Menendez J, Solano RM, et al, Susceptibility to rotenone is increased in neurons from parkin null mice and is reduced by minocycline. *J Neurochem* 2006; **97**: 934–46.

155. Seppi K, Peralta C, Diem-Zangerl A, et al. Placebo-controlled trial of riluzole in multiple system atrophy. *Eur J Neurol* 2006; **13**(10): 1146–8.

156. Koellensperger M, Wenning KG. Parkinson Plus disorders. In: *Therapeutics of Parkinson`s disease and other movement disorders*. Hallet M, ed. Chichester: Wiley Blackwell, 2008; 157–274.

157. Boesch SM, Wenning GK, Ransmayr G, et al. Dystonia in multiple system atrophy. *J Neurol Neurosurg Psychiatry* 2002; **72**: 300–3.

158. Lees AJ, Bannister R. The use of lisuride in the treatment of multiple system atrophy with autonomic failure (Shy–Drager syndrome). *J Neurol Neurosurg Psychiatry* 1981; **44**(4): 347–51.

159. Heinz A, Wöhrle J, Schöls L, et al. Continuous subcutaneous lisuride infusion in OPCA. *J Neural Transm Gen Sect* 1992; **90**(2): 145–50.

160. Goetz CG, Tanner CM, Klawans HL. The pharmacology of olivopontocerebellar atrophy. *Adv in Neurol* 1984; **41**: 143–8.

161. Klos KJ, Bower JH, Josephs KA, et al. Pathological hypersexuality predominantly linked to adjuvant dopamine agonist therapy in Parkinson's disease and multiple system atrophy. *Parkinsonism Relat Disord* 2005; **11**: 381–6.

162. Colosimo C, Merello M, Pontieri FE. Amantadine in parkinsonian patients unresponsive to levodopa: a pilot study. *J Neurol* 1996; **243**(5): 422–5.

163. Wenning GK. Placebo-controlled trial of amantadine in multiple-system atrophy. *Clin Neuropharmacol* 2005; **28**: 225–7.

164. Friess E, Kuempfel T, Modell S, et al. Paroxetine treatment improves motor symptoms in patients with multiple system atrophy. *Parkinsonism Relat Disord* 2006; **12**: 432–7.

165. Lang AE, Lozano A, Duff J, et al. Medial pallidotomy in late-stage Parkinson's disease and striatonigral degeneration. *Adv Neurol* 1997; **74**: 199–211.

166. Visser-Vandewalle V, Temel Y, Colle H, et al. Bilateral high-frequency stimulation of the subthalamic nucleus in patients with multiple system atrophy – parkinsonism. Report of four cases. *J Neurosurg* 2003; **98**: 882–7.

167. Lezcano E, Gomez-Esteban JC, Zarranz JJ, et al. Parkinson's disease-like presentation of multiple system atrophy with poor response to STN stimulation: a clinicopathological case report. *Mov Disord* 2004; **19**: 973–7.

168. Santens P, Vonck K, De Letter M, et al. Deep brain stimulation of the internal pallidum in multiple system atrophy. *Parkinsonism Relat Disord* 2006; **12**(3): 181–3.

169. Jain S, Dawson J, Quinn NP, et al. Occupational therapy in multiple system atrophy: a pilot randomized controlled trial. *Mov Disord* 2004; **19**: 1360–4.

170. Muller J, Wenning GK, Wissel J, et al. Botulinum toxin treatment in atypical parkinsonian disorders associated with disabling focal dystonia. *J Neurol* 2002; **249**: 300–4.

171. Thobois S, Broussolle E, Toureille L, et al. Severe dysphagia after botulinum toxin injection for cervical dystonia in multiple system atrophy. *Mov Disord* 2001; **16**: 764–5.

172. Mancini F, Zangaglia R, Cristina S, et al. Double-blind, placebo-controlled study to evaluate the efficacy and safety of botulinum toxin type A in the treatment of drooling in parkinsonism. *Mov Disord* 2003; **18**: 685–8.

173. Lagalla G, Millevolte M, Capecci M, et al. Botulinum toxin type A for drooling in Parkinson's disease: a double-blind, randomized, placebo-controlled study. *Mov Disord* 2006; **21**: 704–7.

174. Schrag A, Geser F, Stampfer-Kountchev M, et al. Health-related quality of life in multiple system atrophy. *Mov Disord* 2006; **21**: 809–15.

175. Shannon JR, Diedrich A, Biaggioni I, et al. Water drinking as a treatment for orthostatic syndromes. *Am J Med* 2002; **112**(5): 355–60.

176. Young TM, Mathias CJ. The effects of water ingestion on orthostatic hypotension in two groups of chronic autonomic failure: multiple system atrophy and pure autonomic failure. *J Neurol Neurosurg Psychiatry* 2004; **75**: 1737–41.

177. Eichhorn TE, Oertel WH. Macrogol 3350/electrolyte improves constipation in Parkinson's disease and multiple system atrophy. *Mov Disord* 2001; **16**: 1176–7.

178. Jankovic J, Gilden JL, Hiner BC, et al. Neurogenic orthostatic hypotension: a double-blind, placebo-controlled study with midodrine. *Am J Med* 1993; **95**: 38–48.

179. Low PA, Gilden JL, Freeman R, et al. Efficacy of midodrine vs placebo in neurogenic orthostatic hypotension. A randomized, double-blind multicenter study. Midodrine Study Group. *JAMA* 1997; **277**: 1046–51.

180. Mathias CJ, Senard JM, Braune S, et al. L-threo-dihydroxyphenylserine (L-threo-DOPS; droxidopa) in the management of neurogenic orthostatic hypotension: a multi-national, multi-center, dose-ranging study in multiple system atrophy and pure autonomic failure. *Clin Auton Res* 2001; **11**: 235–42.

181. Kaufmann H, Saadia D, Voustianiouk A, et al. Norepinephrine precursor therapy in neurogenic orthostatic hypotension. *Circulation* 2003; **108**: 724–8.

182. Alam M, Smith G, Bleasdale-Barr K, et al. Effects of the peptide release inhibitor, octreotide, on daytime hypotension and on nocturnal hypertension in primary autonomic failure. *J Hypertens* 1995; **13**: 1664–9.

183. Raimbach SJ, Cortelli P, Kooner JS, et al. Prevention of glucose-induced hypotension

by the somatostatin analogue octreotide (SMS 201–995) in chronic autonomic failure: haemodynamic and hormonal changes. *Clin Sci* (Lond) 1989; **77**: 623–8.

184. Halaska M, Ralph G, Wiedemann A, et al. Controlled, double-blind, multicentre clinical trial to investigate long-term tolerability and efficacy of trospium chloride in patients with detrusor instability. *World J Urol* 2003; **20**: 392–9.

185. Sakakibara R, Hattori T, Uchiyama T, et al. Are alpha-blockers involved in lower urinary tract dysfunction in multiple system atrophy? A comparison of prazosin and moxisylyte. *J Auton Nerv Syst* 2000; **79**: 191–5.

186. Mathias CJ, Fosbraey P, da Costa DF, et al. The effect of desmopressin on nocturnal polyuria, overnight weight loss, and morning postural hypotension in patients with autonomic failure. *Br Med J* (Clin Res Ed) 1986; **293**: 353–4.

187. Perera R, Isola L, Kaufmann H. Effect of recombinant erythropoietin on anemia and orthostatic hypotension in primary autonomic failure. *Clin Auton Res* 1995; **5**: 211–13.

188. Winkler AS, Marsden J, Parton M, et al. Erythropoietin deficiency and anaemia in multiple system atrophy. *Mov Disord* 2001; **16**: 233–9.

189. Zesiewicz TA, Helal M, Hauser RA. Sildenafil citrate (Viagra) for the treatment of erectile dysfunction in men with Parkinson's disease. *Mov Disord* 2000; **15**: 305–8.

190. Hussain IF, Brady CM, Swinn MJ, et al. Treatment of erectile dysfunction with sildenafil citrate (Viagra) in parkinsonism due to Parkinson's disease or multiple system atrophy with observations on orthostatic hypotension. *J Neurol Neurosurg Psychiatry* 2001; **71**: 371–4.

191. Iranzo A, Santamaria J, Tolosa E, et al. Long-term effect of CPAP in the treatment of nocturnal stridor in multiple system atrophy. *Neurology* 2004; **63**: 930–2.

192. Ghorayeb I, Bioulac B, Tison F. Sleep disorders in multiple system atrophy. *J Neural Transm* 2005; **112**: 1669–75.

193. Nonaka M, Imai T, Shintani T, et al. Non-invasive positive pressure ventilation for laryngeal contraction disorder during sleep in multiple system atrophy. *J Neurol Sci* 2006; **247**: 53–8.

194. Wenning GK, Pramstaller PP, Ransmayr G, et al. [Atypical Parkinson syndrome]. *Nervenarzt* 1997; **68**(2): 102–15.

195. Colosimo C. Pisa syndrome in a patient with multiple system atrophy. *Mov Disord* 1998; **13**(3): 607–9.

196. Wenning GK, Geser F, Poewe W. The risus sardonicus of multiple system atrophy. *Mov Disord* 2003; **18**: 1211.

Progressive supranuclear palsy

Carlo Colosimo, Giovanni Fabbrini, Alfredo Berardelli

Historical review

Although the earlier literature contained several accounts of progressive supranuclear palsy (PSP) [1], including the famous case reported by Charcot in the nineteenth century [2], the first detailed description of this condition came from John Clifford Richardson, John Steele, and Jerzy Olszewski in the early 1960s [3]. The term PSP was introduced by the same Canadian investigators in 1964 [4]. They described a pre-senile sporadic neurodegenerative disease characterized clinically by a combination of supranuclear vertical ophthalmoplegia, pseudobulbar palsy, nuchal dystonia, and dementia. In their report they described the clinical features of nine patients and reported the neuropathological changes in seven of them. The predominant pathological changes were cell loss and gliosis in the brainstem, basal ganglia, and cerebellum.

In 1986, Pollock and colleagues first reported that the filamentous aggregates found in the brains of patients with PSP shared antigenic determinants with microtubule-associated protein tau [5]. Histopathological studies then confirmed that PSP is a tauopathy characterized by hyperphosphorylated tau protein deposition forming fibrillary aggregates (globose neurofibrillary tangles) in neurons and glia of numerous cerebral areas including the cerebral neocortex, pallidum, subthalamic nucleus, substantia nigra, periacqueductal gray matter, superior collicula, and dentate nucleus [6]. The abundant presence of these aggregates in all clinical PSP subtypes suggested that PSP should be considered a tauopathy along with corticobasal degeneration (CBD), frontotemporal dementia (FTD), and Alzheimer's disease (AD) [7].

The introduction of clinical diagnostic criteria, first proposed by Lees in 1987, made it easier to identify these patients clinically [8]. Others subsequently proposed different sets of diagnostic criteria, mainly based on personal experience [9–11]. New clinical diagnostic criteria were developed in 1996 during a workshop held under the auspices of the National Institute for Neurological Disorders and Stroke and the Society for PSP (NINDS-SPSP) [12]. This time the criteria were also validated on a clinical data set from autopsy-confirmed cases of PSP. Although the NINDS-SPSP criteria (Table 4.1) have gained wide acceptance in the research community and in movement disorder clinics, they remain to be validated prospectively.

Morphological features

Macroscopic examination of the brain in PSP usually shows midbrain atrophy and substantia nigra depigmentation, sometimes with mild frontal lobe atrophy. Microscopic examination

Handbook of Atypical Parkinsonism, eds. Carlo Colosimo, David E. Riley, and Gregor K. Wenning. Published by Cambridge University Press. © Cambridge University Press 2011.

Table 4.1 NINDS/SPSP criteria

Basic features

- gradually progressive disorder
- onset age >40 yr
- no evidence of other diseases that could explain the clinical features as indicated by exclusion criteria*

Diagnosis of clinically possible PSP

- vertical supranuclear palsy#

OR

- slowing of vertical saccades

AND

- postural instability with falls within a year of disease onset

Diagnosis of clinically probable PSP

- vertical supranuclear palsy

AND

- prominent postural instability with falls within a year of disease onset

#Upward gaze is considered abnormal when pursuit or voluntary gaze, or both, have a restriction of ≥50% of the normal range

Supportive features
- symmetrical akinesia or rigidity, proximal more than distal
- abnormal neck posture, especially retrocollis
- poor or absent response of parkinsonism to levodopa
- early dysphagia and dysarthria
- early onset of cognitive impairment including two or more of the following: apathy, impairment in abstract thought, decreased verbal fluency, utilization or imitation behavior, or frontal release signs

*Exclusion criteria**
- recent history of encephalitis
- alien limb syndrome
- cortical sensory deficits
- focal frontal or temporoparietal atrophy
- hallucinations or delusions unrelated to dopaminergic therapy
- cortical dementia of Alzheimer type
- prominent, early cerebellar symptoms
- unexplained dysautonomia
- neuroradiological evidence of relevant structural abnormality
- Whipple's disease, confirmed by polymerase chain reaction

Reproduced with kind permission from Litvan *et al.* [12]

invariably discloses neuronal loss, gliosis, neurofibrillary tangles (NFTs), and neuropil threads (NTs) in the basal ganglia and brainstem. PSP is now considered a tauopathy, characterized by hyperphosphorylated tau protein aggregates. Tau protein binds to microtubules, and plays an important role in neuronal cytoskeletal stability. Alternative splicing of exons 2, 3, and 10 of the tau gene generates six tau isoforms. The inclusion or exclusion of exon 10 produces isoforms with four (4R) or three (3R) microtubule binding sites. Normal brains have similar levels of 4R and 3R, but in some neurodegenerative disorders this ratio is changed. The revised neuropathological criteria for PSP require high NFT and NT densities in at least three of the following brain areas: striatum, oculomotor complex, medulla, or dentate nucleus [13]. The pathological changes often involve the neocortex, especially the primary motor area of the frontal lobe, and severe cell loss in this area has been indicated as a possible contributor to the early falls [14].

In addition to their clinical similarities, PSP and CBD share certain pathological features. This clinicopathological overlap led some to consider the two diseases as different ends of the same disease spectrum. A neuropathological finding of tau-positive tufted astrocytes is considered highly characteristic of PSP and differentiates it from CBD. These astrocytic alterations probably reflect the main degenerative process rather than a change secondary to gliosis. The ballooned neurons typically found in CBD are rarely observed in PSP. The tau aggregates in PSP and CBD contain mainly 4R isoforms and accumulate in neuronal and glial cells. How these aggregates form and how they affect different regions of the brain remain unclear. Ultrastructural examination shows that PSP NFTs consist of mainly straight filaments, whereas AD NFTs contain paired helical filaments [15].

Genetics

The importance of tau aggregates in causing PSP receives further support from genetic findings. PSP is strongly associated with a specific haplotype in the tau gene (denoted as H1). Several reports from different populations show that patients with PSP (like those with CBD) show the H1 haplotype and the H1/H1 genotype significantly more frequently than controls [16]. Fine-mapping of this region detected a variation in a single intron regulating tau expression on the H1 background [17]. A genome-wide association study subsequently discovered a second major susceptibility locus on chromosome 11 that contains several interesting candidate genes [18].

Although PSP is usually a sporadic disease, some studies describe familial clustering. One pedigree with autosomal dominant PSP has been described and linked to a locus on chromosome 1q31, but the gene responsible for the disease in this family still has to be identified [19]. Although mutations in the tau gene may occasionally give rise to a clinical and pathological picture similar to PSP [20,21], screening of large cohorts of sporadic and familial PSP cases has failed to identify tau gene mutations to date.

Clinical picture

Presenting features

The most frequently reported symptom at disease onset is balance problems, followed by personality changes, bulbar symptoms, and visual problems. PSP patients present with a peculiar akinetic-rigid motor disorder that in most cases differs from that observed in Parkinson's disease (PD). Symptoms are more prominent in the axial segments whereas the limbs are relatively preserved [8]. Unlike the onset symptoms in PD, postural stability is compromised early on. In the classic PSP phenotype (recently re-named Richardson's Syndrome, RS), the motor disorder usually responds poorly to levodopa. The poor motor response to dopaminergic drugs is helpful in differentiating between the classic PSP phenotype and PD [22]. A subgroup of PSP patients may nevertheless show a good, but usually short-lived, response to levodopa (PSP-Parkinsonism [PSP-P]) [22]. In some patients, behavioral (apathy, disinhibition) and cognitive (progressive aphasia, apraxia of speech, memory loss) disorders may also be the presenting feature or accompany the motor disorder at disease onset.

Core characteristics of the disease

Patients with PSP generally manifest parkinsonian signs characterized by bradykinesia, rigidity, and disequilibrium with severe gait unsteadiness. The marked axial rigidity influences the posture, which may be characteristically erect like the original cases described by Richardson and colleagues (who described it as "nuchal dystonia," Figure 4.1) or more closely resembles the flexed posture typical of PD. Progressive imbalance leads to repeated and frequent falls (usually backward). Postural tremor and less commonly tremor at rest may be superimposed occasionally. Even so, a classical pill-rolling resting tremor has been reported in less than 20% of the subjects [23]. Patients with PSP frequently have dysphagia and a characteristic growling high-pitched severe dysarthria, with mixed spastic and parkinsonian features [4]. PSP patients also manifest eyelid movement disorders, including blepharospasm and eyelid opening and-closing apraxia. Although neurological examination in patients with PSP sometimes shows pyramidal signs, obvious spastic paraparetic gait or significant pyramidal weakness should cast doubt on the clinical diagnosis of PSP.

The most specific diagnostic feature of PSP is a limitation of vertical gaze with preserved oculocephalic reflexes (Figure 4.2), and many specialists consider frank gaze limitations indispensable for a diagnosis of PSP. Abnormalities of vertical gaze may be absent in up to 50% of the cases, however, and are not often the presenting symptom of PSP [12]. Because some limitation of upgaze is a frequent accompaniment of normal ageing and may be seen in a number of neurodegenerative disorders, limitation of downgaze is a much more specific finding suggestive of PSP. Patients with PSP may also present with other oculomotor disorders (Table 4.2) [24]. The oculomotor disorders are the main component of the peculiar facial expression (often described as worried or astonished) found

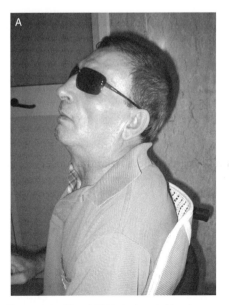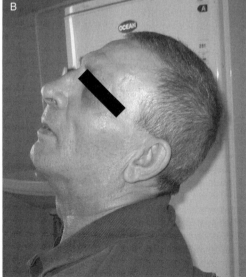

Figure 4.1. (A) and (B) Marked nuchal (neck extensor) dystonia in a patient with probable progressive supranuclear palsy.

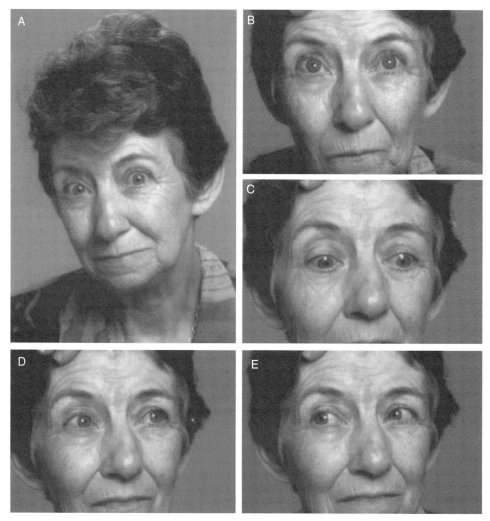

Figure 4.2 Vertical supranuclear ophthalmoplegia with preserved horizontal eye movements in a patient with classical progressive supranuclear palsy.

in patients with PSP, together with the characteristic dystonic features of the frontalis, procerus, and corrugator muscles [25]. The physician needs to differentiate PSP from the numerous other neurological conditions that can initially manifest with oculomotor dysfunction [26–29] (Table 4.3).

Clinical variants

In addition to RS, other clinical syndromes known to accompany PSP-tau pathology include PSP-P (the second most frequent after RS), corticobasal syndrome (CBS) [30], and pure akinesia with gait freezing (PAGF) [31]. These syndromes differ in their clinical features at disease onset and with disease progression. Patients with RD also have a shorter disease course than those with PSP-P and PAGF.

Table 4.2 Oculomotor abnormalities in progressive supranuclear palsy

Early stages

- Slowness of vertical saccadic movements
- Hypometric saccades
- Reduced blinking
- Square wave jerks

Middle stages

- Supranuclear vertical gaze palsy
- Lid retraction with very rare blinking (<3)
- Impaired convergence
- Apraxia of eyelid opening or closing

Late stages

- Supranuclear horizontal gaze palsy
- Loss of oculocephalic reflexes
- Blepharospasm
- Disconjugate gaze

Modified from Golbe [24]

Table 4.3 Other causes of supranuclear ophthalomoplegia associated with parkinsonism

PD
MSA-P
CBD
DLB
FTD and parkinsonism linked to chromosome 17
Huntington's disease
Motor neuron disease
Genetic cerebellar ataxias (SCA 2, SCA 3, SCA 7, SCA 17)
Postencephalitic parkinsonism
Prion diseases
Progressive external ophthalmoplegia
Tumors compressing the brainstem (pinealoma, glioma)
Multi-infarct state
Myasthenia gravis
CNS lymphoma
Niemann–Pick type C disease
Drug-induced
Whipple's disease
Calcification of the basal ganglia

The concept of PSP-P has evolved notably over the past 40 years. The literature repeatedly refers to occasional cases of pathologically definite PSP whose neurological signs and disease course resemble that of PD. Only in recent years, however, did the large clinicopathological series reported by Williams *et al.* [22] underline that this clinical presentation of PSP is far more common than previously recognized. These authors first proposed designating this clinical disease phenotype PSP-P; this form may account for up to one-third of all cases of PSP. Patients with PSP-P typically present with tremor at rest, unilateral or asymmetrical bradykinesia, and a discrete or good response to levodopa. The initial clinical features are difficult to distinguish from those of PD. Multiple system atrophy of the parkinsonian type (MSA-P), particularly in patients without signs of full-blown dysautonomia, may be quite difficult to differentiate clinically from PSP-P [32].

Clinical diagnostic criteria

In 1996, an International Consensus Workshop under the auspices of NINDS and SPSP was convened to develop optimized criteria for a clinical diagnosis of PSP [12]. These diagnostic criteria have since been widely used in the research community and in movement disorder clinics. They define three diagnostic categories of increasing certainty: possible, probable, and definite. The diagnosis of possible and probable PSP depends primarily on the presence of specific clinical features (Table 4.1) and also on exclusion criteria. A definite diagnosis requires a typical PSP neuropathological lesion pattern with tau-positive inclusions.

A retrospective evaluation of the NINDS-SPSP criteria and of the other existing sets of clinical diagnostic criteria for PSP was conducted by Osaki *et al.* [33] on 60 pathologically proven cases from the Queen Square Brain Bank for Neurological Disorders in London. The main features of these diagnostic criteria are summarized in Table 4.4. The diagnosis was made by 40 different physicians on 60 cases clinically diagnosed as PSP when last assessed in life. In 47 cases (78%), the diagnosis of PSP was confirmed pathologically. The findings from this study showed that most cases of PSP were correctly diagnosed by neurologists at the final assessment. Although applying the category "possible," NINDS-SPSP marginally improved the accuracy of the initial clinical diagnosis; none of the existing operational criteria could significantly improve the accuracy of the final clinical diagnosis. All published criteria have good positive predictive values whereas sensitivity is relatively poor [33]. In conclusion, although these formal diagnostic criteria are important for certain clinical

Table 4.4 Outline of features required by different sets of diagnostic criteria for progressive supranuclear palsy

	Gaze abnormalities	Falls	Axial rigidity	Pseudobulbar palsy	Parkinsonism	Frontal lobe signs	LD response
NINDS-SPSP	Vertical	<1 yr	–	–	–	–	–
Lees	Down	Backward	+	+	Brady/rigidity	+	–
Golbe	Down	Not specified	+	+	Brady	–	–
Tolosa	Down	Not specified	+	+	Brady	+	+
Blin	Vertical	Not specified	–	+	Brady/rigidity	–	+

NINDS-SPSP, National Institute for Neurological Disorders and Stroke-Society for Progressive Supranuclear Palsy; LD, levodopa; brady, bradykinesia.
+ or – means that these features are/are not required for diagnosing PSP
Reproduced with kind permission from Osaki et al. [33]

research fields, they add little to the problem of detecting early cases and screening tools need improving.

Time course of the disease

PSP affects both genders, despite a slight male predominance. The disease progresses relentlessly and has a significantly shorter mean survival than PD [24]. The clinical symptoms commonly begin in the seventh decade, although occasionally as early as the fifth decade. Pooling several PSP case series yielded a median onset age of 63 years, with rare cases beginning as early as 40 years of age.

PSP is a chronically progressive disease characterized by the gradual onset of neurological symptoms with increasing disability. In a comparative clinicopathological study, latencies to onset of falls were short in patients with PSP, intermediate in MSA, dementia with Lewy bodies (DLB) and CBD, and long in PD [34]. Recurrent falls within the first year after disease onset predicted PSP in 68% of the patients. Conversely, latency to onset, but not duration, of recurrent falls differentiates PD from other examples of parkinsonism. In another study, the progression to different Hoehn and Yahr (HY) stages was evaluated in 81 pathologically confirmed patients with parkinsonism. Latencies to each HY stage were longer in patients with PD than in those with atypical parkinsonism (AP). Development of a HY-III within one year of motor onset accurately predicted AP. The progression to each HY stage was unhelpful in distinguishing the various disorders with AP from each other. Once patients with PD and AP became wheelchair-bound, both had equally short survival times [35].

The prognosis of PSP remains poor. This is a progressive disorder associated with a shortened life span, often leading to death within ten years after symptom onset. Mean survival ranges from 5.9 to 9.7 years according to the different series.

Epidemiology

The dearth of published epidemiological studies makes it difficult to determine incidence and prevalence rates for PSP. The estimated prevalence of PSP (per 100 000 in the population) in the various studies ranged from 1.3 to 4.9 [36,37]. The estimated annual incidence of PSP was about 0.3–1.1 cases per 100 000 persons or 5.3/100 000 people over the age of 50 years [38]. These figures match those for other well-known neurodegenerative disorders such as Huntington's disease or motor neuron disease. The analytical epidemiology of PSP is even poorer and more controversial. Although a retrospective study conducted in Switzerland showed an increased risk of PSP associated with arterial hypertension [39] other independent series failed to confirm the finding [40]. Smoking habits seem to be similar to those in healthy controls. The fact that the inverse association with smoking found previously in PD is shared by MSA but not by PSP lends epidemiological support to the notion that different smoking habits are associated with different groups of neurodegenerative disease [41].

Investigations

Introduction

The clinical diagnosis of PSP depends primarily on history and physical examination. Recent evidence, however, shows that additional investigations may be useful in differentiating PSP from other parkinsonian syndromes.

Computerized tomography

Although CT scans sometimes disclose pathological changes including generalized or brainstem atrophy in patients with PSP, current data suggest that this diagnostic tool is of limited use in routine clinical practice [8].

Routine magnetic resonance imaging

Several studies have sought to improve the diagnostic accuracy of PSP by using various MRI techniques [42]. Routine and volumetric MRI imaging may show midbrain atrophy, a finding that helps in differentiating patients with PSP from healthy controls and those with PD and other disorders with AP. A study designed to provide a quantitative assessment of atrophy by measuring midbrain diameter or area found that a diameter of <17 mm on axial MRIs differentiates patients with PSP from healthy controls [43]. Other studies suggest that atrophy is better evaluated on mid-sagittal slices because they are not subject to variation in the scanning angle. The midbrain atrophy seen on these slices typically resembles a penguin or hummingbird silhouette [44]. In a study designed to measure the midbrain area in patients with PSP, Japanese investigators found a significant area reduction in PSP versus PD and controls [45]. The relationship between the midbrain/pons areas was also significantly lower in patients with PSP than that observed in PD patients and controls. Although these measurements were helpful in differentiating PSP, MSA, and PD as groups, the data obtained overlapped among the groups of patients investigated, and therefore were not helpful for an individual diagnosis.

In a study investigating morphometric MRI in PSP, MSA, PD, and controls using volumetric T1-weighted sequences [46], Quattrone and colleagues measured the midbrain and pons areas, together with the medial cerebellar peduncle (MCP) and superior cerebellar peduncle (SCP) width. They found that atrophy in PSP involves the midbrain and SCP whereas atrophy in MSA involves the the pons and the MCP. In patients with PD all brain areas measured had dimensions similar to those in control subjects. Single structure measurements did not discriminate among the different diseases on an individual basis, because of substantial overlap. The investigators therefore proposed a new index calculated with a specific formula (area of pons/area of midbrain x MCP diameter/SCP diameter) obtained by combining the single measurements obtained in the various cerebral structures. The 'magnetic resonance parkinsonism index' (MRPI) was significantly higher in PSP than in the other conditions, and could differentiate individual patients with PSP from those with MSA and PD. The promising results obtained with morphome tric MRI should be confirmed in studies conducted by other groups before proposing its use in routine clinical practice.

Diffusion-weighted imaging

Diffusion-weighted imaging (DWI) is a useful diagnostic tool that can provide additional support for a diagnosis of AP, and especially for PSP. In their study, Seppi and coworkers found significantly higher rADC (regional apparent diffusion coefficient) values in both the putamen and globus pallidus in patients with PSP than in those with PD [47]. The increased putaminal rADC values in PSP probably reflect ongoing striatal degeneration, whereas most neuropathological studies reveal an intact striatum in PD. Despite these differences, increased putaminal rADC values are not able to discriminate PSP from MSA-P.

Magnetic resonance volumetry

Whether magnetic resonance volumetry will help in differentiating PSP from other disorders with AP remains to be confirmed. Patients with PSP, MSA-P, and MSA-C had significantly lower mean striatal and brainstem volumes than patients with PD, and patients with MSA-P and MSA-C also showed a reduction in cerebellar volume [48]. Total intracranial volume-normalized MRI-based volumetric measurements also provide a sensitive marker to discriminate PD from AP.

Voxel-based morphometry is an observer-unbiased volumetric procedure that can be used to investigate the entire brain. A study comparing patients with probable PSP and healthy controls showed that in patients with PSP several cortical areas in the frontal, temporal, and insular lobes were decreased in volume [49]. White matter comparisons also disclosed a volume reduction in the frontotemporal regions and the mesencephalon. This brain atrophy pattern probably accounts for the cardinal PSP-associated behavioral deficits.

Functional imaging

Functional imaging methods for differential diagnosis in AP are techniques designed to investigate receptor binding and glucose metabolism. Studies of brain receptor binding in parkinsonism, by evaluating dopa-decarboxylase activity and the dopamine transporter (DAT) examine the presynaptic nigrostriatal neurons, and by evaluating the dopamine D2-receptors examine postsynaptic dopaminergic function. More recently, SPECT and PET ligands have become available to study cardiac sympathetic innervation.

Using PET, the Hammersmith group found that putaminal uptake of the presynaptic dopaminergic marker ^{18}F-fluorodopa was reduced to a similar extent in PD and PSP [50]; in some patients with PSP, caudate uptake was also markedly reduced, as opposed to only a moderate reduction in PD [51]. Measurements of striatal dopamine D2-receptor densities using raclopride and PET also failed to differentiate between PD and AP, demonstrating a similar loss of densities in patients with advanced PD, PSP, and MSA [52].

SPECT evaluation of DAT using ^{123}I-β-CIT may be useful in differentiating true parkinsonism from patients with essential tremor and patients with parkinsonism owing to a subcortical vascular encephalopathy. Although PSP cannot be distinguished from PD with this method alone [53], patients with PSP may show a more symmetrical DAT loss, consistent with the more symmetrical clinical motor dysfunction observed in this condition. SPECT imaging studies of patients with dopa-naïve parkinsonism have used ^{123}I-IBZM as a D2-receptor ligand [54]. Subjects with normal IBZM binding responded well to apomorphine and benefitted from subsequent chronic dopaminergic therapy, whereas subjects with reduced binding failed to respond. In some of these patients, other clinical features atypical for PD developed during follow-up [55]. Despite these interesting findings, because striatal IBZM binding is also reduced in other disorders with AP such as MSA, IBZM binding has limited predictive value for an early diagnosis of PSP [56].

Scintigraphic visualization of postganglionic sympathetic cardiac neurons was found to differentiate patients with PD from patients with AP [57]. Considering all reports published so far, standard scintigraphy with ^{123}I-metaiodobenzylguanidine (MIBG), a technique used for years to detect pheochromocytoma cells, correctly distinguished most patients with PD, all of whom had severely reduced cardiac MIBG uptake. This radioactive ligand method appears to be a highly sensitive and specific tool to discriminate between PD and AP within two years after the onset of symptoms but it cannot distinguish PSP from other forms of AP such as MSA [58].

Neurophysiology

Among the standard neurophysiological tests used in patients with abnormal eye movements, electro-oculographic recording may help in distinguishing patients with PSP from those with CBD at an early stage [59]. Patients with PSP have decreased horizontal saccadic amplitude and velocity but normal latency, whereas those with CBD show normal saccadic velocity and increased latency. The antisaccadic task (looking in the direction opposite to a visual stimulus), which correlates well with frontal lobe dysfunction, is markedly impaired in patients with PSP, although it may also be impaired in AD. Conversely, patients with PD or MSA-P have no or only slight saccadic impairment [60].

In a recent study by our group, when we recorded blink movements in patients with PSP we found that voluntary, spontaneous, and reflex blinking all show abnormal kinematic features, also observing a correlation between abnormal kinematic variables and patients' clinical features [61]. Our findings suggest that abnormal blinking in patients with PSP reflects the widespread cortical, subcortical, and brainstem degenerative changes related to this disease.

Other neurophysiological measures of brainstem function are abnormal, reflecting the pathological alterations in the midbrain and pons typical of PSP. An absent or a severely reduced startle reaction has been described in patients with PSP, whereas it was only mildly affected in PD patients [62]. The orbicularis oculi response to an electrical stimulus is abnormal in patients with PSP in whom electrical median-nerve stimulation elicits a normal mentalis response [59]. These findings differentiate patients with PSP from those with PD, MSA, and CBD, in whom peripheral nerve stimulation invariably elicits simultaneous responses in the orbicularis oculi and mentalis muscles.

In patients with parkinsonism, diagnostic neurophysiological studies now commonly include external anal or urethral sphincter EMG. Owing to degeneration of Onuf's nucleus, the anal and urethral external sphincter muscles both undergo denervation and re-innervation [63]. Neurogenic changes in the sphincter muscles can be present in patients with PSP [64]. Sphincter EMG recordings nevertheless have limited diagnostic value in PSP because they almost invariably disclose similar abnormalities in patients with MSA as well [65]. Another disadvantage of sphincter-EMG recordings is confounding from non-specific abnormalities such as chronic constipation, previous pelvic surgery, or vaginal deliveries [66].

Finally, although somatosensory, visual, and brainstem evoked potentials are usually normal in PSP, the presence of abnormal motor potentials evoked by transcranial magnetic stimulation and a prolonged central motor conduction time suggests the involvement of pyramidal tracts. In addition, PSP patients show an increased cortical excitability as demonstrated by an abnormal input–output curve [67].

Other investigations

Although several studies over the past 15 years have sought PSP biomarkers in cerebrospinal fluid (CSF), none of them has provided findings that can be applied in clinical practice. For example, Holmberg and colleagues [68] first showed that the CSF neurofilament (NFL) content was significantly higher in patients with PSP and MSA than in those with PD, reflecting the degree of ongoing neuronal degeneration affecting mainly the axonal compartment. They also proposed that combining CSF-NFL dosing and a levodopa test may improve the differential diagnosis of parkinsonian syndromes [69]. Whereas the CSF-NFL test predicted 79% and levodopa tests predicted 85% correct diagnoses (PD vs. non-PD [MSA and PSP]), the combined test predicted 90% correct diagnoses.

CSF levels of total tau protein in patients with PSP were found to be similar to those in controls and patients with AD [70], but significantly increased in patients with CBD. In contrast, in fact a recent study found that patterns of proteolytic tau fragments in CSF from patients with PSP differed from those in patients with other neurodegenerative conditions such as AD, FTD, CBD, and PD [71]. These results using qualitative tau-measures are promising, and if confirmed by other groups may indicate a possible biomarker for diagnosing patients with PSP early in the disease course.

Treatment

Given the few randomized controlled studies so far conducted, the symptomatic management of PSP is based largely on empirical evidence.

General approach

A number of therapeutical approaches, other than pharmacological, are important in PSP: for example, physical therapy, speech therapy, occupational therapy, and psychological support for patients and carers; macrogol-water solution [72] for constipation; and food thickeners, feeding via a nasogastric tube, or percutaneous endoscopic gastrostomy for dysphagia. (See also Chapter 8). These management decisions should be based on careful clinical judgment, taking into account the patient's and caregivers' expectations.

Treatment of parkinsonism

Most patients with PSP have parkinsonian features and these should be a major target for therapeutic intervention. Unfortunately, dopaminergic treatment provides only modest results. Open-label or retrospective studies suggest that up to 30% of patients with PSP may benefit from levodopa at least transiently [22]. Occasionally, a beneficial effect is evident only when seemingly unresponsive patients deteriorate after levodopa withdrawal. Results with dopamine agonists have been even more disappointing [24]. Anti-parkinsonian effects have been reported in a few patients with PSP treated with amantadine but an open study including subjects with PSP reported no significant improvement [73].

Treatment of other clinical features

PSP involves the dopaminergic and also the cholinergic systems [74]. Unfortunately, studies with the cholinesterase inhibitor donepezil found no improvement in the cognitive dysfunction associated with this disease [75]. Blepharospasm, apraxia of eyelid opening, scialorrhea, as well as limb and nuchal dystonia may respond well to local injections of botulinum toxin A [76].

Neuroprotection trials

Despite the disappointing results from the first trials with coenzyme Q10 [77] and riluzole [78], several international groups are conducting multicenter intervention trials with possible disease-modifying agents in PSP. These trials should change our approach to PSP. For example, they will provide previously unavailable prospective data concerning disease progression that can be used to identify reliable predictors of survival.

In addition, a specific rating instrument has recently been developed to standardize severity assessments in specialized clinics and research programs worldwide [79]. The PSP rating scale (PSPRS) is a prospectively validated clinical tool that represents a convenient global measure of disability and disease progression in PSP. The score on this disease-specific scale increases at a rate of around 10 points per year in patients with clinically probable PSP, up to a maximum of 100 points. This new tool will be helpful for planning future phase III intervention trials more effectively during the next decade.

Conclusions

The recently obtained molecular information along with findings from clinical trials of disease-modifying agents hopefully should bring about a major change in our therapeutic approach to this devastating illness.

References

1. Brusa A, Stoehr R, Pramstaller PP. Progressive supranuclear palsy: new disease or variant of postencephalitic parkinsonism? *Mov Disord* 2004; **19**: 247–52.
2. Goetz CG. An early photographic case of probable progressive supranuclear palsy. *Mov Disord* 1996; **11**: 617–8.
3. Richardson JC, Steele JC, Olszewski J. Supranuclear ophthalmoplegia, pseudobulbar palsy, nuchal dystonia and dementia. *Trans Am Neurol Assoc* 1963; **8**: 25–9.
4. Steele JC, Richardson JC, Olszewski J. Progressive supranuclear palsy. A heterogeneous degeneration involving the brain stem, basal ganglia and cerebellum with vertical gaze and pseudobulbar palsy, nuchal dystonia and dementia. *Arch Neurol* 1964; **10**: 333–59.
5. Pollock NJ, Mirra SS, Binder LI, et al. Filamentous aggregates in Pick's disease, progressive supranuclear palsy, and Alzheimer's disease share antigenic determinants with microtubule-associated protein, tau. *Lancet*; 2(8517): 1211.

6. Daniel SE, de Bruin V, Lees AJ. The clinical and pathological spectrum of Steele-Richardson-Olszewski syndrome (progressive supranuclear palsy): a reappraisal. *Brain* 1995; **118**: 759–70.
7. Williams DR. Tauopathies: classification and clinical update on neurodegenerative diseases associated with microtubule-associated protein tau. *Intern Med J* 2006; **36**: 652–60.
8. Lees AJ. The Steele–Richardson–Olszewski syndrome (progressive supranuclear palsy). In: Marsden CD, Fahn S, eds. *Movement disorders 2*. London: Butterworths, 1987; 272–87.
9. Blin J, Baron JC, Dubois B, et al. Positron emission tomography study in progressive supranuclear palsy. Brain hypometabolic pattern and clinicometabolic correlations. *Arch Neurol* 1990; **47**: 747–52.
10. Golbe LI, Davis PH. Progressive supranuclear palsy. In: Jankovic J, Tolosa E, eds. *Parkinson's disease and movement disorders*. Baltimore: Williams and Wilkins, 1993; 145–61.
11. Tolosa E, Valldeoriola F, Marti MJ. Clinical diagnosis and diagnostic criteria of progressive supranuclear palsy

(Steele-Richardson-Olszewski syndrome). *J Neural Transm Suppl* 1994; **42**: 15–31.

12. Litvan I, Agid Y, Calne D, et al. Clinical research criteria for the diagnosis of progressive supranuclear palsy (Steele-Richardson-Olszewski syndrome): report of the NINDS-SPSP International Workshop. *Neurology* 1996; **47**: 1–9.

13. Hauw JJ, Daniel SE, Dickson D, et al. Preliminary NINDS neuropathologic criteria for Steele-Richardson-Olszewski syndrome (progressive supranuclear palsy). *Neurology* 1994; **44**: 2015–9.

14. Halliday GM, Macdonald V, Henderson JM. A comparison of degeneration in motor thalamus and cortex between progressive supranuclear palsy and Parkinson's disease. *Brain* 2005; **128**: 2272–80.

15. Montpetit V, Clapin DF, Guberman A. Substructure of 20 nm filaments of progressive supranuclear palsy. *Acta Neuropathol* 1985; **68**: 311–18.

16. Bennett P, Bonifati V, Bonuccelli U, et al. Direct genetic evidence for involvement of tau in progressive supranuclear palsy. European Study Group on Atypical Parkinsonism Consortium. *Neurology* 1998; **51**: 982–5.

17. Rademakers R, Melquist S, Cruts M, et al. High-density SNP haplotyping suggests altered regulation of tau gene expression in progressive supranuclear palsy. *Hum Mol Genet* 2005; **14**: 3281–92.

18. Melquist S, Craig DW, Huentelman MJ, et al. Identification of a novel risk locus for progressive supranuclear palsy by a pooled genomewide scan of 500,288 single-nucleotide polymorphisms. *Am J Hum Genet* 2007; **80**: 769–78.

19. Ros R, Gomez GP, Hirano M, et al. Genetic linkage of autosomal dominant progressive supranuclear palsy to 1q31.1. *Ann Neurol* 2005; **57**: 634–41.

20. Pastor P, Pastor E, Carnero C, et al. Familial atypical progressive supranuclear palsy associated with homozygosity for the delN296 mutation in the tau gene. *Ann Neurol* 2001; **49**: 263–7.

21. Morris HR, Osaki Y, Holton J, et al. Tau exon 10+16 mutation FTDP-17 presenting clinically as sporadic young onset PSP. *Neurology* 2003; **61**: 102–4.

22. Williams DR, de Silva R, Paviour DC, et al. Characteristics of two distinct clinical phenotypes in pathologically proven progressive supranuclear palsy: Richardson's syndrome and PSP-parkinsonism. *Brain* 2005; **128**: 1247–58.

23. Collins SJ, Ahlskog JE, Parisi JE, et al. Progressive supranuclear palsy: neuropathologically based diagnostic clinical criteria. *J Neurol Neurosurg Psychiatry* 1995; **58**: 167–73.

24. Golbe LI. Progressive supranuclear palsy. In: Beal M Flint, Lang AE, Ludolph A, eds. *Neurodegenerative diseases.* Cambridge: Cambridge University Press, 2005; 663–81.

25. Romano S, Colosimo C. Procerus sign in progressive supranuclear palsy. *Neurology* 2001; **57**: 1928.

26. van Zagten M, Lodder J, Kessels F. Gait disorder and parkinsonian signs in patients with stroke related to small deep infarcts and white matter lesions. *Mov Disord* 1998; **13**: 89–95.

27. Siderowf AD, Galetta SL, Hurtig HI, et al. Posey and Spiller and progressive supranuclear palsy: an incorrect attribution. *Mov Disord* 1998; **13**: 170–4.

28. Averbuch-Heller L, Paulson GW, Daroff RB, et al. Whipple's disease mimicking progressive supranuclear palsy: the diagnostic value of eye movement recording. *J Neurol Neurosurg Psychiatry* 1999; **66**: 532–5.

29. Campdelacreu J, Kumru H, Tolosa E, et al. Progressive supranuclear palsy syndrome induced by clebopride. *Mov Disord* 2004; **19**: 482–4.

30. Boeve BF, Maraganore DM, Parisi JE, et al. Pathologic heterogeneity in clinically diagnosed corticobasal degeneration. *Neurology* 1999; **53**: 795–800.

31. Riley DE, Fogt N, Leigh RJ. The syndrome of 'pure akinesia' and its relationship to progressive supranuclear palsy. *Neurology* 1994; **44**: 1025–9.

32. Colosimo C, Albanese A, Hughes AJ, et al. Some specific clinical features differentiate multiple system atrophy (striatonigral variety) from Parkinson's disease. *Arch Neurol* 1995; **52**: 294–8.

33. Osaki Y, Ben-Shlomo Y, Lees AJ, et al. Accuracy of clinical diagnosis of

progressive supranuclear palsy. *Mov Disord* 2004; **19**: 181–9.

34. Wenning GK, Ebersbach G, Verny M, et al. Progression of falls in postmortem-confirmed parkinsonian disorders. *Mov Disord* 1999; **14**: 947–50.

35. Müller J, Wenning GK, Jellinger K, et al. Progression of Hoehn and Yahr stages in parkinsonian disorders: a clinicopathologic study. *Neurology* 2000; **55**: 888–91.

36. Chio A, Magnani C, Schiffer D. Prevalence of Parkinson's disease in northwestern Italy: comparison of tracer methodology and clinical ascertainment of cases. *Mov Disord* 1998; **13**: 400–5.

37. Schrag A, Ben-Shlomo Y, Quinn NP. Prevalence of progressive supranuclear palsy and multiple system atrophy: a cross-sectional study. *Lancet* 1999; **354**: 1771–5.

38. Bower JH, Maraganore DM, McDonnell SK, et al. Incidence of progressive supranuclear palsy and multiple system atrophy in Olmsted County, Minnesota, 1976 to 1990. *Neurology* 1997; **49**: 1284–8.

39. Ghika J, Bogousslavsky J. Presymptomatic hypertension is a major feature in the diagnosis of progressive supranuclear palsy. *Arch Neurol* 1997; **54**: 1104–8.

40. Colosimo C, Osaki Y, Vanacore N, et al. Lack of association between progressive supranuclear palsy and arterial hypertension: a clinicopathological study. *Mov Disord* 2003; **18**: 694–7.

41. Vanacore N, Bonifati V, Fabbrini G, et al. Smoking habits in multiple system atrophy and progressive supranuclear palsy. *Neurology* 2000; **54**: 114–19.

42. Olanow CW. Magnetic resonance imaging in parkinsonism. *Neurol Clin* 1992; **10**: 405–20.

43. Schrag A, Good CD, Miszkiel K, et al. Differentiation of atypical parkinsonian syndromes with routine MRI. *Neurology* 2000; **54**: 697–702.

44. Kato N, Arai K, Hattori T. Study of the rostral midbrain atrophy in progressive supranuclear palsy. *J Neurol Sci* 2003; **210**: 57–60.

45. Oba H, Yagishita A, Terada H, et al. New and reliable MRI diagnosis for progressive supranuclear palsy. *Neurology* 2005; **64**: 2050–5.

46. Quattrone A, Nicoletti M, Messina D, et al. MR imaging index for differentiation of progressive supranuclear palsy from Parkinson disease and the Parkinson variant of multiple system atrophy. *Radiology* 2008; **246**: 214–21.

47. Seppi K, Schocke MFH, Esterhammer R, et al. DWI discriminates PSP from PD, but not from the Parkinson variant of multiple system atrophy, *Neurology* 2003; **60**: 922–7.

48. Schulz JB, Skalej M, Wedekind D, et al. Magnetic resonance imaging-based volumetry differentiates idiopathic Parkinson's syndrome from multiple system atrophy and progressive supranuclear palsy. *Ann Neurol* 1999; **45**: 65–74.

49. Brenneis C, Seppi K, Schocke M, et al. Voxel based morphometry reveals a distinct pattern of frontal atrophy in progressive supranuclear palsy. *J Neurol Neurosurg Psychiatry* 2004; **75**: 246–9.

50. Brooks DJ, Ibanez V, Sawle GV, et al. Differing patterns of striatal 18-F-Dopa uptake in Parkinson`s disease, multiple system atrophy and progressive supranuclear palsy. *Ann Neurol* 1990; **28**: 547–55.

51. Burn DJ, Sawle GV, Brooks DJ. Differential diagnosis of Parkinson's disease, multiple system atrophy, and Steele-Richardson-Olszewski syndrome: discriminant analysis of striatal 18F-dopa PET data. *J Neurol Neurosurg Psychiatry* 1994; **57**: 278–84.

52. Brooks DJ, Ibanez V, Sawle GV, et al. Striatal D2 receptor status in patients with Parkinson's disease, striatonigral degeneration, and progressive supranuclear palsy, measured with 11C-raclopride and positron emission tomography. *Ann Neurol* 1992; **31**: 184–92.

53. Brücke T, Asenbaum S, Pirker W, et al. Measurement of the dopaminergic degeneration in Parkinson's disease with [123I] beta-CIT and SPECT. Correlation with clinical findings and comparison with multiple system atrophy and progressive supranuclear palsy. *J Neural Transm Suppl* 1997; **50**: 9–24.

54. Schwarz J, Tatsch K, Arnold G, et al. 123I-iodobenzamide-SPECT in 83 patients with

de novo parkinsonism. *Neurology* 1993;
43: 17–20.

55. Schwarz J, Tatsch K, Gasser T, et al.
123I-IBZM binding compared with
long-term clinical follow-up in patients
with de novo parkinsonism. *Mov Disord*
1998; **13**: 16–19.

56. van Royen E, Verhoeff NF, Speelman
JD, et al. Multiple system atrophy
and progressive supranuclear palsy.
Diminished striatal D2 dopamine receptor
activity demonstrated by 123I-IBZM single
photon emission computed tomography.
Arch Neurol 1993; **50**: 513–16.

57. Orimo S, Ozawa E, Nakade S, et al. (123)
I-metaiodobenzylguanidine myocardial
scintigraphy in Parkinson's disease.
J Neurol Neurosurg Psychiatry 1999;
67: 189–94.

58. Yoshita M. Differentation of idiopathic
Parkinson's disease from striatonigral
degeneration and progressive
supranuclear palsy using iodine-123
meta-iodobenzylguanidine myocardial
scintigraphy. *J Neurol Sci* 1998; **155**: 60–7.

59. Valls-Solé J. Neurophysiological aids to
the diagnosis of progressive supranuclear
palsy (PSP). *Suppl Clin Neurophysiol* 2006;
58: 249–56.

60. Vidailhet M, Rivaud S, Gouider-Khouja
N, et al. Eye movements in parkinsonian
syndromes. *Ann. Neurol* 1994; **35**: 420–6.

61. Bologna M, Agostino R, Gregori B, et al.
Voluntary, spontaneous and reflex blinking
in patients with clinically probable
progressive supranuclear palsy. *Brain* 2009;
132: 502–10.

62. Vidailhet M, Rothwell JC, Thompson PD,
et al. The auditory startle response in the
Steele-Richardson-Olszewski syndrome
and Parkinson's disease. *Brain* 1992;
115: 1181–92.

63. Palace J, Chandiramani VA, Fowler CJ.
Value of sphincter electromyography in
the diagnosis of multiple system atrophy.
Muscle Nerve 1997; **20**: 1396–403.

64. Valldeoriola F, Valls-Sole J, Tolosa ES,
et al. Striated anal sphincter denervation
in patients with progressive supranuclear
palsy. *Mov Disord* 1995; **10**: 550–5.

65. Vodusek D. Sphincter EMG and
differential diagnosis of multiple system
atrophy. *Mov Disord* 2001; **16**: 600–7.

66. Colosimo C, Inghilleri M, Ray Chaudhuri K.
Parkinson's disease misdiagnosed as
multiple system atrophy by sphincter
electromyography. *J Neurol* 2000;
247: 559–61.

67. Kühn AA, Grosse P, Holtz K, et al. Patterns
of abnormal motor cortex excitability in
atypical parkinsonian syndromes. *Clin
Neurophysiol* 2004; **115**: 1786–95.

68. Holmberg B, Rosengren L, Karlsson JE,
et al. Increased cerebrospinal fluid levels
of neurofilament protein in progressive
supranuclear palsy and multiple-system
atrophy compared with Parkinson's
disease. *Mov Disord* 1998; **13**: 70–7.

69. Holmberg B, Johnels B, Ingvarsson P, et al.
CSF-neurofilament and levodopa tests
combined with discriminant analysis may
contribute to the differential diagnosis of
Parkinsonian syndromes. *Parkinsonism
Relat Disord* 2001; **8**: 23–31.

70. Urakami K, Mori M, Wada K, et al. A
comparison of tau protein in cerebrospinal
fluid between corticobasal degeneration
and progressive supranuclear palsy.
Neurosci Lett 1999; **259**: 127–9.

71. Borroni B, Gardoni F, Parnetti L, et al.
Pattern of tau forms in CSF is altered in
progressive supranuclear palsy. *Neurobiol
Aging* 2009; **30**: 34–40.

72. Eichhorn TE, Oertel WH. Macrogol
3350/electrolyte improves constipation in
Parkinson's disease and multiple system
atrophy. *Mov Disord* 2001; **16**: 1176–7.

73. Colosimo C, Merello M, Pontieri FE.
Amantadine in parkinsonian patients
unresponsive to levodopa: a pilot study.
J Neurol 1996; **243**: 422–5.

74. Juncos JL, Hirsch EC, Malessa S, et al.
Mesencephalic cholinergic nuclei in
progressive supranuclear palsy. *Neurology*
1991; **41**: 25–30.

75. Fabbrini G, Barbanti P, Bonifati V, et al.
Donepezil in the treatment of progressive
supranuclear palsy. *Acta Neurol Scand*
2001; **103**: 123–5.

76. Ward AB, Molenaers G, Colosimo C,
et al. Clinical value of botulinum toxin
in neurological indications. *Eur J Neurol*
2006; **13**(Suppl 4): 20–6.

77. Stamelou M, Reuss A, Pilatus U, et al.
Short-term effects of coenzyme Q10 in
progressive supranuclear palsy: a

randomized, placebo-controlled trial. *Mov Disord* 2008; **23**: 942–9.

78. Bensimon G, Ludolph A, Agid Y, et al. NNIPPS Study Group. Riluzole treatment, survival and diagnostic criteria in Parkinson plus disorders: the NNIPPS study. *Brain* 2009; **132**: 156–71.

79. Golbe LI, Ohman-Strickland PA. A clinical rating scale for progressive supranuclear palsy. *Brain* 2007; **130**: 1552–65.

Chapter 5

Corticobasal degeneration

Melissa J. Armstrong and Anthony E. Lang

Introduction and history

While historical review suggests earlier reports of the entity now known as corticobasal degeneration (CBD), the disease was first clearly described in a series of three cases in 1968, when it was termed corticodentatonigral degeneration with neuronal achromasia [1]. Subsequent terminology has included corticonigral degeneration with neuronal achromasia [2], corticobasal ganglionic degeneration [3], cortical-basal ganglionic degeneration [4], and corticobasal degeneration [5]. While the more precise terminology of cortical-basal ganglionic degeneration (CBGD) may be favored, the most commonly used descriptor today is CBD.

As understanding of this complex disease process has grown over the forty years since the original clinicopathological series, it has become clear that the corticobasal spectrum involves a clinical syndrome and a pathological entity that only sometimes overlap (Figure 5.1). Because of this, the clinical diagnosis is now labeled the corticobasal syndrome (CBS) while the term CBD is reserved for pathologically confirmed diagnoses [6]. As will be discussed further, the pathological entity of CBD is associated with varying clinical presentations that can change even in a single individual over time, while CBS is associated with a variety of findings on pathological examination. It is only in this context that the current understanding of CBD can be discussed. The overlap of CBS, CBD, and related disorders is considerable, making accurate clinical diagnosis challenging and emphasizing the need for continued research.

Because CBD is a pathological diagnosis, discussion of this entity must begin with neuropathological findings. CBD is a sporadic neurodegenerative process related to abnormal aggregation of hyperphosphorylated tau. Tau is a microtubule-associated protein the role of which in the neuron is to promote microtubule assembly and stabilization. Other tauopathies include frontotemporal dementia with parkinsonism linked to chromosome 17 (FTDP-17), progressive supranuclear palsy (PSP), and Pick's disease (PiD). In particular, CBD is associated with abnormal insoluble tau isoforms with four conserved repeat sequences (4R tau), discussed further in the following sections.

The Office of Rare Diseases published criteria for CBD in 2002 (Table 5.1). The criteria emphasize the presence of tau-immunoreactive lesions in addition to the presence of ballooned neurons, cortical atrophy, and nigral degeneration [7]. Diagnosis is based on histopathological findings, although gross findings can provide supportive information. Confirmation of the diagnosis requires identification of the pathological features of CBD

Handbook of Atypical Parkinsonism, eds. Carlo Colosimo, David E. Riley, and Gregor K. Wenning. Published by Cambridge University Press. © Cambridge University Press 2011.

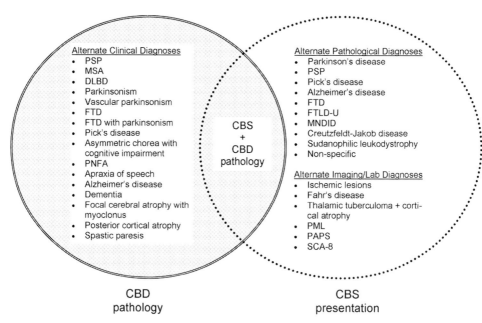

Figure 5.1 The spectrum of corticobasal degeneration.

and the exclusion of other pathologies, such as those associated with Alzheimer's disease (AD) and Lewy body disorders [7]. Familial cases (often with much younger onset than typical sporadic cases) with identical neuopathological features may be a result of FTDP-17 associated with specific mutations in the tau gene.

The cardinal clinical features of CBS, initially described with this CBD pathology, are no longer felt to be pathognomonic for this disease. CBD is thus a pathological diagnosis with varying clinical presentations.

Epidemiology

CBD is a rare neurodegenerative disease and its exact incidence and prevalence are unknown. In a series of 143 patients with parkinsonism seen at a movement disorders center and proceeding to autopsy, four (2.8%) were diagnosed neuropathologically with CBD. Those patients who had neuropathological assessment, however, represented only approximately 8% of patients admitted to the hospital for parkinsonism and less than 5% of patients attending outpatient clinics [8]. By assuming that CBD accounts for approximately 1% of patients diagnosed clinically with parkinsonism at movement disorders clinics and estimating the number of diagnoses that might be missed, the incidence of CBD has been estimated at 0.62/100 000 to 0.92/100 000 and prevalence in the United States has been estimated at 13 000 to 20 000 [9].

Pathology

As discussed in the introduction of this chapter, neuropathological criteria for CBD emphasize the histopathological findings of tau-immunoreactive lesions in addition to ballooned neurons, cortical atrophy, and nigral degeneration (Table 5.1) [7]. The ballooned

Table 5.1 Office of Rare Diseases neuropathological criteria for the diagnosis of corticobasal degeneration

Core features
Neuronal and glial lesions with tau pathology demonstrated by Gallyas stain or tau immunostaining
• Thread-like lesions and astrocytic plaques in gray and white matter
• Prominent tau immunoreactivity in cell processes
Caudate and putamen involvement with tau-immunoreactive lesions
Moderate to marked neuronal loss in the substantia nigra
Cortical neuronal loss and astrogliosis
• Most cortical pathology is in the superior frontal, superior parietal, and pre- and post-central gyri
Supportive features
Gross findings
• Narrowing of cortical gyri, most prominently in parasagittal regions, often peri-Rolandic
• Cortical atrophy, particularly in the posterior frontal lobe
• Cortical spongiosis
• Thinning of the corpus callosum
• Flattening of the caudate head and small thalamic volume
• Pale substantia nigra
Swollen, "achromatic," or "ballooned" neurons
Neurofibrillary lesions in brainstem monoaminergic nuclei (e.g. locus ceruleus and substantia nigra) (previously called "corticobasal bodies")
Oligodendroglial tau-positive argyrophilic inclusions, sometimes named "coiled bodies"
Sparing of hippocampus and parahippocampal gyrus
Exclusion criteria*
Senile plaques and Alzheimer-type neurofibrillary tangles
Classic Pick's bodies with sharply defined margins
Lewy bodies, α-synuclein pathology
Ubiquitin immunoreactivity
Infarcts, hemorrhages, and/or focal ischemic damage

* Cases are sometimes described as "mixed" pathologies, which can display these findings (mixed cases must also meet criteria for the coexistent diagnosis)

Adapted from Dickson et al. [7]

achromatic neurons, which were once emphasized as a major component of the histopathology and gave the disorder its original name, are now believed to be non-specific, seen in varying numbers in many other neurodegenerative disorders and closely resembling Pick's cells of PiD.

The Office of Rare Diseases notes that the pathology found in some patients can be mixed, with features of both CBD and other disorders, usually also neurodegenerative in nature. To classify a mixed pathological diagnosis, the autopsy findings must fully meet the criteria for CBD and for the pathological diagnosis that coexists [7]. Schneider *et al.* reported that 6 of 11 CBD cases manifested neuropathological overlap; coexistent disorders included AD, PSP, Parkinson's disease (PD), and hippocampal sclerosis [10]. Other studies have also emphasized overlap with AD, PSP, synucleinopathies, and argyrophilic grain disease [11–13]. One study found that only 2 of 8 CBD cases had pure CBD pathology [12]. In a recent review of neuropathological findings in a series of PSP patients, 32% of the cases reviewed showed coexistent CBD changes [14].

Central to the diagnosis of CBD is the presence of abnormal tau aggregations, seen by special staining of pathological specimens. Tau is typically considered a neuronal microtubule-associated protein. However, its presence is also now recognized in astrocytes and oligodendrocytes [15]. Six tau isoforms are found in human adult brains, resulting from alternative splicing patterns. The variations in splicing of exon 10 generate isoforms containing either three (3R-tau) or four (4R-tau) microtubule-binding repeats. Normal adult human brains express approximately equal levels of 3R-tau and 4R-tau, but this ratio is changed in pathological processes, such as when mutations disrupt normal exon 10 splicing [16]. Most cases of CBD are thought to be associated with up-regulation of 4R-tau containing exon 10 [16]. In both CBD and PSP, 4R-tau accumulations are prominent in the cerebral cortices while basal ganglia and brainstem accumulations are immunopositive for 4R-tau and occasionally 3R-tau [15].

Abnormal tau immunoreactivity is found in both the neurons and the glia. In neurons, tau immunohistochemistry reveals diffuse or granular cytoplasmic staining, pretangles, and small neurofibrillary tangles. These probably account for the corticobasal inclusions found in subcortical gray matter regions including the substantia nigra. Tau immunoreactive threads in both neurons and glia are numerous in gray and white matter. CBD pathology includes astrocytic plaques with tau deposition largely in the distal processes of astrocytes. These astrocytic plaques are distinct from tufted astrocytes found in PSP, where tau is deposited more proximally to the cell body as well as in distal processes. While CBD and PSP both demonstrate oligodendroglial inclusions, coiled bodies, and threads, the astrocytic changes can distinguish the two diagnoses [7,15]. In addition, while threads are numerous and diffuse in CBD, they are rarely seen in the cerebral cortices in PSP, although they may be dense in other areas [17].

A recent neuropathological study has discovered the presence of TAR-DNA-binding protein 43 (TDP-43) in a subset of patients with CBD pathology. TDP-43 is a protein pathologically deposited in the disorder currently termed frontotemporal lobar degeneration with ubiquitin-positive inclusions and TDP-43-immunoreactive inclusions (FTLD-U) as well as in amyotrophic lateral sclerosis (ALS). In 15.4% of CBD cases, TDP-43-positive inclusions were seen in various patterns. TDP-43 pathology was also seen in 25.8% of AD cases, but was not found in PiD or PSP [18]. There was no clear clinical correlation with the presence of TDP-43 inclusions in CBD. The significance of the findings remains unclear other than highlighting the overlap between CBD, CBS, and FTLD-U, discussed further in the following sections.

Genetics

CBD is generally considered a sporadic disorder, although a small number of families with apparent autosomal dominant inheritance have been described. However, it is now recognized that certain inherited mutations in the tau gene can result in pathology identical to that of sporadic CBD; for example, P301L [19] and N296N [20,21] mutations (with or without the CBS clinical phenotype described later in the chapter). Other tau mutations, to date lacking pathological correlation, can result in a familial CBS; for example, P301S [22] and

G289R mutations [23]. There is no consensus in the literature as to whether these cases should be classified primarily as CBD owing to defined mutations or as FTDP-17 with CBD-like pathology. The failure to identify a mutation in one family may be related to the use of archival rather than fresh samples [24]. Another family without a defined mutation had one member with CBD pathology and a sibling with PSP pathology, suggesting an underlying tau process distinct from that in sporadic CBD [25].

Although no tau mutations have been found in sporadic CBD to date, evidence does support involvement of the tau gene. An analysis of tau polymorphisms in CBD has shown that the frequencies of H1 tau haplotypes and H1/H1 genotypes are significantly higher in patients with CBD compared to controls [26]. All seven CBD cases in a separate report similarly demonstrated the H1 haplotype and H1/H1 genotype [12]. The H1 tau haplotype has also been associated with PSP [26], suggesting a common genetic predisposition to these two disorders. In a recent evaluation of patients with clinical pictures suggestive of PSP, CBS, or combined PSP and CBS, the haplotype found was H1 in over 90% of each of the three subgroups [27].

In patients with sporadic and familial CBS, the most common genetic causes found are mutations in the gene coding for the protein progranulin (*PRGN*) [13,28–32]. Neuropathological findings in these patients are more consistent with FTLD-U rather than CBD. In addition to tau and PRGN mutations, other genetic causes of a CBS have included a sporadic spinocerebellar ataxia mutation (SCA-8) [33] and a hereditary prion protein mutation in a large family where one of the individuals was diagnosed with CBS [34]. Consistent with the diverse genetic processes underlying CBS as compared to CBD, tau haplotype studies have shown both association of CBS with certain tau haplotypes [35] and lack of such an association [36].

Animal models

No widely studied animal models of CBD currently exist. Various worm, fly, and mouse models for tauopathies have been used to study this class of diseases in general and are well described in a recent review [37]. Certain transgenic mouse models are more appropriate for consideration in CBD than others. CBD neuropathology is most notable for the presence of astrocytic plaques and prominent tau-positive neuropil threads. Thus, those models producing similar tau-related pathological changes may be more appropriate for ongoing study in the context of CBD [38–40].

Clinical findings

Initial reports of CBD described hallmark clinical features including asymmetric disease, parkinsonism, tremor, limb dystonia, gait abnormalities, myoclonus, alien limb phenomena, cortical sensory loss, and apraxia [1,2,4,5,41]. Only a small number of patients in each of these series had pathological correlations.

Since the initial descriptions, it has become clear that the clinical syndrome of CBS does not correlate reliably with CBD. While the pathology may reveal CBD, patients meeting clinical criteria for CBS also have a wealth of other neuropathological diagnoses including PD [8], PSP [42–46], PiD [43–47], AD [6,44,48,49], frontotemporal dementia (FTD) without distinctive histopathology [8], FTLD-U [13,31,32] including motor neuron disease inclusion dementia (MNDID) [50], Creutzfeldt-Jakob disease (CJD) [44,51–53], sudanophilic leukodystrophy [43], and non-specific pathology (Figure 5.1). Because of the relative rarity of CBD, it is difficult to calculate the positive predictive value of a premortem diagnosis of CBS as has been done for other disorders with parkinsonism.

In addition to presentations of CBS, discussed further in the following sections, patients with CBD have demonstrated clinical features overlapping with many other disorders. Various clinical presentations and diagnoses have been described in patients with CBD pathology (Figure 5.1), including clinical syndromes mistaken for PSP [8,13,45,54–56], multiple system atrophy (MSA) [13,56], diffuse Lewy body disease (DLBD) [56], non-specific parkinsonism [8,56], FTD [12,13,45,57,58], PiD [13,56], chorea [57], AD and other dementias [13,56,57,59], and spastic paresis [60]. PSP, FTD, and progressive non-fluent aphasia (PNFA) are the most common non-CBS clinical presentations reported with CBD.

In the next section, first discussed are the clinical features reported in classical CBS (often lacking confirmatory pathology) and then the clinical features reported in patients proven to have CBD at postmortem examination are reviewed.

Corticobasal syndrome

The core features of CBS are a progressive asymmetrical akinetic-rigid syndrome and associated higher cortical signs, most prominently apraxia [4,41,61,62].

Movement disorders

CBS is an atypical parkinsonism. Symptoms typically start unilaterally, with the arm more commonly affected at presentation than the leg [41]. Common initial complaints include clumsiness, incoordination, stiffness, or jerking of the affected arm [41,62]. On examination, this limb is typically found to be akinetic, rigid, and apraxic, sometimes associated with dystonia [41]. In a predominantly clinical series, 95% of patients had at least two of the parkinsonian signs of bradykinesia, rigidity, tremor, and gait disorder [61]. The initial involvement of one arm tends to progress over two years, with subsequent involvement of the contralateral arm or the ipsilateral leg and eventually general disability [62]. The parkinsonism of CBS characteristically fails to respond to levodopa and this has been suggested as a possible diagnostic criterion for the disease [61–63].

While tremor can be present and has been reported in 30–55% of patients with CBS [61,64], the tremor tends to be different from that seen in idiopathic PD [61]. It may begin as a postural and action tremor and only rarely has a resting element. It is often jerky in appearance [62]. Semi-rhythmic bursts of myoclonus can falsely give the appearance of a tremor at rest. The tremor may progress to myoclonus [62].

Movement disorders other than the classic asymmetrical akinetic-rigid syndrome are also common in CBS. Dystonia is present in 59–71% of individuals in various series mixing cases of clinical and pathological diagnoses [4,61,64]. In a study of 36 patients with CBS, 33% had dystonia at the initial evaluation, but 83% had dystonia at their last follow-up [41]. Dystonia is present often at rest rather than being purely action-induced. Typically, the dystonia affects the involved arm and hand at onset [41,62,64], with 92% of CBS patients with dystonia exhibiting upper limb involvement [64]. When symptoms begin in the leg, dystonic inversion of the foot can be seen [62], with 28% of CBS patients with dystonia developing leg involvement [64]. The head, neck, and trunk are less often involved. In a series looking specifically at dystonia in CBS, 74% of the patients with dystonia developed associated fixed postures and 42% had accompanying pain, most commonly in a dystonic hand [64].

Myoclonus has been reported in 55–93% of patients with CBS [4,41,61,64]. As mentioned, the myoclonus may evolve from a postural tremor. It tends to be action- and stimulus-induced and involves the distal arm, often in association with dystonia. Here the dystonia at rest may result in myoclonus not associated with voluntary activation of the limb. Rarely, a similar presentation can be seen in the leg [62,65,66].

Other movement disorders occurring in association with CBS include athetosis and oro-lingual dyskinesia [4,64]. Postural instability and falls are more common later in the disease course and are often multifactorial, related to parkinsonism, dystonia, and lower limb apraxia. In the rarer cases where leg involvement is prominent at onset, instability may occur earlier [62].

Higher cortical dysfunction

In addition to the akinetic-rigid syndrome, higher cortical signs are a classic component of the CBS picture, present in 93% of patients [61]. These include apraxia, alien limb phenomena, cortical sensory loss, frontal lobe reflexes, dementia, and aphasia [4,61]. Apraxia is the most common higher cortical finding in most series, with various categories of apraxia seen (Table 5.2). Ideomotor apraxia is the most frequently recognized apraxia in CBS, with some patients demonstrating an overlapping ideational apraxia [67]. Limb-kinetic apraxia has also been reported as the dominant apraxia in CBS [68]. While it is the initially affected limb that typically becomes most profoundly apraxic, the evaluation of this is often hampered by the presence of the dystonia and parkinsonism [62]. To compensate for this, formal evaluation of apraxia has usually been conducted using the limbs least affected by the primary motor disorder [67]. In some patients, symptoms of apraxia can be the presenting complaint, as in the case of a surgeon who first noticed that he had "forgotten" how to glove, tie knots, and use instruments with his left hand [4].

Alien limb phenomena (ALP) are variably present in CBS, occurring in 42–67% of patients [4,41,61,64]. The movements are not always described, however, and debate remains about the proper definition of alien limb behavior [62,69]. Patients may dissociate themselves from the limb, calling the limb "it" and feeling as though it has a mind of its own [62]. Various types of ALP are known (Table 5.3), including intermanual conflict, mirror movements, enabling synkinesis, grasping, impulsive groping, magnetic apraxia, utilization behavior with compulsive manipulation of tools, and purposeless wandering [69]. Attempts have been made to divide ALP into frontal, callosal, and more recently, posterior subtypes, but the validity of these groupings remains unclear [69].

An early series of CBS patients (some with pathologically proven CBD) described ALP as including uncontrollable wandering, grasping behaviors, and interference with the contra-lateral limb, either as a foreign presence or simply out of voluntary control [41]. Involuntary phenomena described in case reports of pathologically-proven CBD include levitation and interference with the other arm's movements [1], involuntary head scratching [2], arm levitation and tentacle-like movements of the fingers [5], uncontrollable repetitive tasks including putting on and taking off glasses and moving tissues in and out of a purse [4], levitation and touching of the lips [4], and elevation, wandering, and spontaneous paddling movements [70]. Bilateral involuntary movements have been reported in two CBD patients: in an early series, one man had levitation of the left hand with touching of the lips and repetitive involuntary movements of the right arm toward the face [4], while a recent report details continuous tactile pursuit with the left hand and a levitating tactile avoidance response with the right hand [71].

Given the parietal localization of signs of higher cortical dysfunction in CBS, it is not surprising that many of the descriptions of ALP in CBS are consistent with the proposed posterior subtype of ALP, where the alien movements tend to appear purposeless and wandering

Table 5.2 Common types of apraxia seen in corticobasal syndrome

Type of apraxia	Definition	Examples
Limb-kinetic apraxia	Inability to make coordinated, fine finger movements	Picking up a coin from a table and rotating a coin in one's hand may be impaired
Ideomotor apraxia	Inability to correctly perform a voluntary movement, demonstrating mistakes in space, posture, and speed of movements	When asked to pantomime movements, patients will make errors. Patients asked to demonstrate use of a "tool" (a transitive gesture) will make errors. For example, when asked to mimic brushing their teeth, they may use their finger to represent a toothbrush rather than moving as if grasping a toothbrush. Spatial and joint movements may also be incorrect. Intransitive gestures (e.g. saluting, snapping fingers) and copied movements may be impaired
Ideational apraxia	Inability to carry out parts of a plan in the proper sequence. Patients may also be unable to identify the use of specific objects	Patients may be unable to identify the use of common objects, such as hammers or can openers. Patients may also do tasks out of order, such as putting a bow on a giftbox before the wrapping paper. This can be tested by giving three-step commands

rather than the more purposeful movements described in frontal and callosal ALP. Simple levitation, however, can be seen in parietal lesions without ALP, which is why one set of proposed research criteria for CBS specifically excluded actions that appear to be simple levitation [63]. Simple levitation is a common source of misdiagnosis in CBS. Personal experience with CBS suggests that compulsive groping and grasping (magnetic apraxia) is a particularly common form of ALP in CBD.

Cortical sensory loss was present in 14 of the 16 patients in an early series and was the sole initial symptom in three of these patients [4]. It was present in 33–59% of patients in other clinical series [41,61,64]. Affected patients often complain of numbness and tingling and some have been treated with inappropriate – and unsuccessful – carpal tunnel release [62]. Examination may reveal normal primary sensory modalities with impaired joint position sense and two-point discrimination. Agraphesthesia and astereognosis may also be present [62].

The prominent presence of cognitive dysfunction in CBD has become increasingly evident; this is discussed further in the following sections. While dementia was initially considered an exclusion criterion for CBS [63], it is now clear that cognitive impairment frequently accompanies CBS. Neuropsychological testing performed in patients with CBS shows global deterioration, executive dysfunction, and impairments in language

Table 5.3 Alien limb phenomena

Behavior	Description	Comment
Intermanual conflict	One hand acts at cross-purposes with the other	Commonly seen with callosal lesions; typically affects non-dominant hand; rare in CBS
Mirror movements	One hand mimics the other hand's movements	
Enabling synkinesis	One hand can do a task only in unison with the other hand	
Magnetic apraxia	Compulsive reaching, groping, and grasping; difficulty releasing objects	Reported in CBS; common in CBS based on personal experience
Utilization behavior	Compulsive handling and using of tools	Reported in CBS
Purposeless movements	Arm wandering, levitation combined with other movements, and other purposeless activities	Commonly seen with posterior lesions; very common in CBS with ALP

and visuospatial functioning [72,73]. Often calculation is also impaired [74]. In general, semantic memory appears to be minimally affected, at least early in the disease course [62,72,73].

Language dysfunction is part of the cortical dysfunction seen in CBS. It has been noted with increased frequency in recent studies, possibly because initially it was overshadowed by prominent motor features [75]. In early reports of CBS, aphasia was reported in 10–21% of cases [4,61]. A review of cognitive processes in CBS subsequently has found aphasia reported in 31% of clinically diagnosed cases [73]. Half of CBS patients studied showed evidence of aphasia syndromes on Western Aphasia Battery testing [75]. In a separate assessment of 10 patients with CBS, only two had clinically apparent aphasia, but the majority showed some degree of language impairment, particularly on phonologic and spelling tests [76]. When present, the aphasia typically is non-fluent or anomic [73,75].

Other clinical manifestations of corticobasal syndrome

In addition to the classic features of a movement disorder with higher cortical dysfunction, patients with CBS are described as having pyramidal findings, impaired ocular motion, impaired eyelid motion, dysarthria, and dysphagia [4,61,64]. Of these, pyramidal signs such as hyperreflexia (often asymmetrical) and extensor plantar responses are the most commonly reported [4,61,62].

Oculomotor abnormalities have been reported in 66.7% of CBS patients [64], requiring differentiation from the closely related PSP. Studies of patients with CBS and clinically diagnosed PSP suggest that CBS patients have equally affected horizontal and vertical eye movements and demonstrate slowed initiation of saccades with markedly increased saccadic latencies. This is in contrast to PSP, where vertical saccades tend to be more affected than horizontal and where the prominent impairment is decreased saccadic velocity rather than abnormal latency [77]. In a recent study examining various clinically diagnosed neurode-generative diseases, vertical oculomotor abnormalities were universally more prominent than those in the horizontal direction. PSP was the only condition that exhibited abnormal saccadic velocity. While PSP showed increased latency only with vertical saccades, CBS and AD showed increased latency with both vertical and horizontal saccades. Saccadic gain was most impaired in the PSP group but was also seen in CBS and AD patients. FTLD subsets showed variable but less prominent oculomotor findings [78].

Case reports describe Balint's syndrome [79], visuomotor ataxia [80], and visual hallucinations [81] occurring within the context of the clinical syndrome of CBS. Impaired smell has been reported recently in a CBS cohort [82]. Depression, and to a lesser extent, apathy, irritability, and agitation, are neuropsychiatric symptoms observed in CBS patients [83]. A combination of spastic dysarthria and pathological laughter and crying was reported as a presenting feature in two women who developed typical features of CBS several years later [84].

The Pick complex

Because of the overlap of the motor symptoms of CBS with cognitive and language dysfunction, and because of the potential for several different pathological disorders to cause CBS, it has been suggested that CBS and CBD be categorized under the broad heading of the Pick complex [45,85–88]. This umbrella term has been proposed to include a number of diagnoses [45,86], most prominently PiD, FTD, primary progressive aphasia (PPA), PNFA, semantic dementia, PSP, and CBS/CBD [45,86,87]. In a series of 60 patients with these clinical diagnoses and subsequent autopsy, 45 had pathology compatible with FTD/Pick complex. Ten of the remaining 15 patients had AD on autopsy and the other five had heterogeneous findings. Of the 45 patients with FTD/Pick complex pathology, 24 had tau-negative pathology and 21 had tau-positive pathology. The most common histological findings were (tau negative) motor neuron disease-type inclusions (40%). CBD was the second most common pathological diagnosis (27%) [87]. Similar findings were reported by a second group, where of 61 patients with clinical variants of FTD, 31 had tau-positive inclusions and 30 had tau-negative neuropathology. Nine patients (15%) were diagnosed with CBD [89].

Within the context of the Pick complex, a concept has been proposed describing the evolution of clinical syndromes over time. Syndromes can be labeled first, second, and third based on the clinical diagnoses for which criteria are met sequentially over time. This concept has been studied in several series from the same group [85,87,88]. The most recent series of 55 patients with CBS showed that of the 19 patients with a motor presentation of CBS, 18 progressed to a second syndrome of either FTD or progressive aphasia (PA). Seven patients then progressed to a third syndrome of either FTD or PA. Of the 36 patients with cognitive onset of CBS, all 15 patients starting with clinical features of FTD progressed to show evidence of both CBS and PA as second and third syndromes in varying orders. Twenty-one patients initially had symptoms of PPA, 12 of whom had both secondary and tertiary syndromes of CBS and FTD and nine of whom only had a secondary syndrome of CBS with no further evolution to a third syndrome at the time of the report. Autopsy findings were available for 19 of these patients, with evidence of CBD, PSP, CBD/PSP mixed pathology, prion disease, PiD, AD, and FTD with motor neuron disease-type inclusions. All patients with CBD demonstrated CBS at some time during the course of their illness, but sometimes not until the later stages [88].

Clinical features of corticobasal degeneration

Three series of patients with pathologically proven CBD describe clinical features of 42 patients [56,59,90]. In the earliest of these series, the presentation was consistent with classic descriptions of CBS. Asymmetric limb clumsiness with or without rigidity (50%) and tremor (21%) were the most common early symptoms. Findings most commonly seen at the initial neurological consultation – an average of three years after symptoms started – were unilateral limb rigidity (79%), bradykinesia (71%), ideomotor apraxia (64%), postural imbalance (45%), unilateral limb dystonia (43%), and cortical dementia (36%) [56].

In the subsequent series, involving 28 patients, early and prominent cognitive dysfunction was more common than the classic motor presentation of CBS. In the series reported by Grimes *et al.*, only 4 of the 13 patients had CBS. Nine patients had early cognitive impairment, six of whom were given the clinical diagnosis of AD. All but 1 of the 13 patients in this series had cognitive dysfunction before death. Five of these patients also had early language dysfunction [59]. In the most recent series, 53.3% of patients with CBD presented solely with a cognitive complaint, 20% presented solely with a motor complaint, and 26.7% presented with mixed complaints. Cognitive complaints involved memory, language, and other cognitive skills. Only six of these patients received a correct diagnosis of CBD before their deaths, five of whom had motor signs on initial testing [90]. In all three series, almost all patients developed at least one extrapyramidal motor sign prior to death [56,59,90].

Neuropsychological testing of CBD patients demonstrates difficulties with learning tasks, word fluency, verbal comprehension, perceptual organization, and cognitive flexibility [57]. Aphasia has been reported in 44% of pathologically diagnosed cases [73], with early language dysfunction present in 29%, 38.5%, and 46.7% of CBD patients in the above series [56,59,90]. The frequency of language dysfunction increases over the course of the disease, with 50–71.4% of patients demonstrating language dysfunction prior to death [56,90]. In one CBD series, language dysfunction – including effortful speech, word-finding difficulties, and/or handwriting difficulty – was the most commonly reported early complaint [90]. Apraxia of speech (AOS) has also been reported both as the sole presenting feature of CBD and in combination with aphasia [70,91], with a recent review emphasizing that a subset of both CBD and PSP patients may have only AOS or PNFA at disease onset without associated parkinsonism [92]. Preliminarily, prominent AOS may be more PSP-related and prominent language dysfunction may be more likely CBD-related, but this association needs further confirmation [92].

CBD patients lacking asymmetrical parkinsonism at onset of disease, especially those presenting with cognitive disturbances, are the most likely to be misdiagnosed. An absence of ideomotor apraxia and the alien limb sign also contribute to misdiagnosis [59,90,93].

The previously discussed concept of first, second, and third syndromes in patients with CBS is obviously relevant to cases where the pathology is proven to be that of CBD. In the series reporting symptom and syndrome progression over time, the ten patients with a pathological diagnosis of pure CBD reflected various orders of syndrome evolution. All ten eventually developed features of CBS. However, only two started with a motor syndrome, both later displaying FTD and PA syndromes. The other eight CBD patients had cognitive presentations. Four began with FTD and four with PA symptoms. All but one patient demonstrated all three syndromes of CBS, FTD, and PA, emphasizing the clinical heterogeneity of the disorder. Half of the ten exhibited CBS as the third syndrome, underscoring that

Table 5.4 Clinical features of corticobasal degeneration

Onset between 45 and 75 years old, most commonly in 50s and 60s

Insidious onset and gradual progression

Early cognitive impairment, often at presentation

- Executive impairment

- Visuospatial impairment

Language abnormalities

- May occur apart from other cognitive impairment

Motor abnormalities

- Parkinsonism, usually asymmetric

- Dystonia, usually asymmetric

- Tremor

- Myoclonus

- Gait abnormalities, usually with late falls

Cortical abnormalities (other than impaired cognition)

- Apraxia

- Alien limb phenomena

- Cortical sensory loss

Absence of response to dopaminergic therapy

motor features may develop only late in the course of CBD [88]. Clinical features of CBD are summarized in Table 5.4.

Other clinical manifestations

In addition to classic CBS features and prominent cognitive impairment, patients with CBD demonstrate varying degrees of pyramidal findings, visual and oculomotor complaints and findings, and depression. Pyramidal findings include hyperreflexia and extensor plantar responses [56,59,94] and may be a source of misdiagnosis [93]. One unusual patient with CBD demonstrated a progressive spastic paraparesis for five years before extrapyramidal signs became evident [60].

Visuospatial complaints have been presenting concerns for patients in multiple CBD series and reports [56,90,94]. Presentation of CBD as a posterior cortical atrophy syndrome results in clinical findings such as homonymous hemianopia, visual neglect, optic ataxia, visual agnosia, and simultagnosia [56,59,90,94]. Apraxia of eyelid opening and abnormalities of oculomotor movements including apraxia of gaze, gaze impersistence, impaired saccades, and supranuclear gaze palsies are also described in CBD [1,4,5,56,59]. Some kind of visuospatial or ocular abnormality is seen in 50–62% of CBD patients prior to death [56,90]. No studies have examined differences in eye movement abnormalities in cases of pathologically proven CBD compared to PSP.

While the presence of neuropsychiatric features has not been assessed formally in CBD, behavior changes are common, as reflected in the overlap with FTD. Depression has been reported in approximately 30% of patients at symptom onset and approximately 40% prior to death [56,90].

Natural history

CBD symptom onset is typically in the sixth and seventh decades of life [4,5,45,56]. Mean ages at onset reported are 60.9, 63, and 63.9 years, with a range of 45–75 years [45,56,90]. CBS has been reported in patients as young as 27 and 28 years old, one case of which was associated with a tau mutation and a positive family history. Neither case had associated neuropathology [22,95]. Presentation at a young age should prompt investigation for tau or PRGN mutations or some other symptomatic cause (e.g. prion disease) rather than assuming a diagnosis of sporadic CBD. Men and women are equally affected by CBD [45,56,59,90].

The onset of CBD is insidious and it is relentlessly progressive [4,41,56,62]. Mean disease duration was 7.9 years and 5.4 years in two pathology series, with ranges of 2.5–12.5 years and 2.0–7.5 years, respectively [56,90]. In a study of the natural history of CBD, statistically significant predictors of shorter survival included first visit findings of bilateral bradykinesia, a frontal syndrome, or the presence of at least two of three extrapyramidal features (tremor, rigidity, or bradykinesia). All patients with available postmortem cause-of-death information died of bronchopneumonia [56].

Investigations

Discussion of investigations for CBD is complicated by the fact that most reports involve primarily patients with CBS without pathological confirmation. This will be re-emphasized throughout the following section. Typically, routine blood, urine, and cerebrospinal fluid (CSF) analyses are normal in CBD. Multiple studies have investigated possible CSF biomarkers in CBS compared to controls and other disorders with parkinsonism, particularly PSP. Researchers have measured CSF tau [96–100], orexin [101], β-amyloid [102], neurofilament heavy chain component [103], and homovanillic acid levels [104]. Levels of CSF tau compared to controls and compared to PSP and other neurodegenerative conditions have been variable and all of these studies are limited by the lack of pathological confirmation, thus allowing for overlap between studied groups. Further studies are needed to determine whether any of these possibilities will be a reliable biomarker for these conditions that require pathological confirmation.

Neuropsychological testing

As discussed in the previous sections, cognitive dysfunction, including aphasia, is common in CBD. Tasks of learning and word fluency were impaired in patients with autopsy diagnoses of CBD and PSP in a recent study; subjects with CBD performed worse on tests of verbal comprehension, perceptual organization, and cognitive flexibility compared to controls [57]. Longitudinal neuropsychological assessments in CBD patients show impaired executive, language, and visuospatial processes with relatively preserved episodic memory. The Mini-Mental State Examination was not sensitive for the deficits found on neuropsychological testing [90].

Patients with CBS have depression (73%), apathy (40%), irritability (20%) and agitation (20%) on the Neuropsychiatric Inventory. General neuropsychological testing has shown the classic asymmetrical apraxias (not surprising, given criteria used for diagnosis) with a dysexecutive syndrome. The cognitive profile of patients with CBS includes a moderate dementia with impaired attention and concentration, verbal fluency, language, and visuospatial tasks but intact semantic memory [72,105].

Neuroimaging

The exact role of neuroimaging in diagnosing CBD is still evolving, but it is useful in ruling out contributory focal lesions, at least. For example, anatomical imaging in patients with clinical pictures overlapping with CBS have occasionally shown focal abnormalities suggestive of ischemic lesions [43], Fahr's disease [106], CJD [52], and a thalamic tuberculoma with associated focal cortical atrophy [107].

Various imaging modalities have been studied in patients with CBS but no pathological confirmation. The most common MRI feature reported in CBS is asymmetrical cortical and cerebral peduncle atrophy, usually contralateral to the clinically more profoundly affected side [108–110]. Posterior frontal and parietal lobes are usually more severely atrophied. Fluid-attenuated inversion recovery (FLAIR) imaging commonly reveals frontal and/or parietal subcortical white matter changes [108], often with subtle peri-rolandic hyperintensities that can be bilateral [108,109]. Mild to moderately severe white matter changes have been described in 40–48% of CBS patients [64]. Basal ganglia changes reported to date have been variable [108,109].

In pathologically proven CBD, MRI scans have shown cortical atrophy, particularly frontal and parietal, and atrophy of the corpus callosum [111,112]. Unlike imaging studies reported in patients with CBS, MRIs in CBD have usually shown relatively symmetrical cortical atrophy [112,113]. Basal ganglia atrophy has also been reported [112]. When CBS patients with CBD pathology were compared to CBS patients with other neurodegenerative pathologies, no features were found to be specific for CBD [111].

Specialized MR techniques such as MRI-based volumetery [113], voxel-based morphometry [110], MR spectroscopy (MRS) [114], and functional MRI [109] have been investigated preliminarily in CBS, but their utility remains unclear.

Two studies have assessed volumetric MRI in CBD. One found that a model combining the midbrain, pons, parietal white matter, temporal gray matter, brainstem, and frontal white matter volumes could differentiate CBD patients from pathologically proven PSP patients and controls, whereas analysis of any one area could not [113]. Voxel-based morphometry also showed differences between CBD and pathologically proven PSP. Semiquantitative analysis in patients with primary extrapyramidal presentations showed that the CBD subgroup had moderate cortical gray matter atrophy and subcortical white matter atrophy while the PSP subgroup had moderate brainstem atrophy. In contrast, CBD patients presenting with prominent cognitive disturbance had severe cortical and moderate subcortical gray matter atrophy with minimal white matter changes, while the PSP patients presenting in this fashion showed moderate cortical gray and subcortical white matter atrophy and mild brainstem and subcortical gray matter atrophy [112].

Positron emission tomography (PET) imaging with [18F]-fluorodeoxyglucose (FDG) in CBS patients shows asymmetrical patterns of glucose metabolism [115–119]. These findings, however, simply corroborate the distribution of the underlying process and provide no insight into the nature of the pathology. PET imaging with [11C](R)-(1-[2-chlorophenyl]-N-methyl-N-[1-methylpropyl]-3-isoquinoline carboxamide) (PK11195), a marker of peripheral benzodiazepine-binding sites expressed by activated microglia, showed that four CBS patients had increased microglial activation in the basal ganglia and cortical regions corresponding to the locations of abnormalities found on typical CBD neuropathological examination [120]. Clinical applications of this finding need to be further elucidated.

CBS SPECT studies show asymmetrical frontoparietal hypoperfusion [108,109] consistent with known localization of clinical findings but without insight into the underlying pathological processes. Striatal fluorodopa uptake studies have shown variable degrees of asymmetry and extent of caudate and putaminal uptake, with reports of both significant and insignificant differences compared to typical PD [116,119,121].

One study of transcranial sonography reported that patients with CBS had marked substantia nigra hyperechogenicity compared to clinically diagnosed PSP patients, but pathological confirmation was lacking for both groups [122].

Electrophysiology

In case reports of CBD where it is mentioned, electroencephalography (EEG) has been normal or has shown slow- and sharp wave activity, particularly over the more affected hemisphere, and/or diffuse bilateral slowing [1,4]. Studies of patients with CBS without pathological confirmation have demonstrated asymmetrical slowing including focal intermittent slow waves (typically contralateral to the dominantly affected limb), intermittent sharp waves, and less commonly, frontal intermittent rhythmic delta activity and slowing of background activity [114,123].

Electrophysiological studies have been used to assess myoclonus in CBS. No electrophysiological studies have been reported of patients with pathologically proven CBD. Electrophysiological testing of the myoclonus in CBS has found a pattern different from other syndromes with parkinsonism and suggestive of a cortical process, although distinct from classic cortical reflex myoclonus [65,124–126]. While most studies suspect a cortical source of the myoclonus, a subcortical origin has also been proposed [127]. Typically, the electromyography (EMG) pattern shows synchronous short duration bursts (20–50 ms) of upper limb muscle discharges (agonist and antagonist muscles) and a lack of associated large EEG potentials or giant somatosensory evoked potentials (SEPs) [65,124–126]. Short latencies (approximately 40 ms) are typically reported between stimulus and elicited jerk [65,124,125]. In addition, the long-latency responses (LLRs) are reported to be enhanced at rest in CBS patients and to have an abnormally increased amplitude during motor activation [125].

Somatosensory evoked potentials are typically but variably abnormal in CBS. Abnormal morphology of the parietal P25-N33 component [65], abnormal morphology of the parietal N20-P25 complex [126], and minimal abnormalities in parietal SEP responses but absent frontal SEP responses [125] have all been reported.

Transcranial magnetic stimulation (TMS) in CBS patients shows variable disruption of the ipsilateral silent period indicating callosal pathology [128]. A study of TMS in various syndromes with parkinsonism showed persistent callosal impairment in both CBS and PSP groups with intact ipsilateral silent periods in MSA and ideopathic PD patients [129]. Recently, normal TMS findings in a patient with CBS supported consideration of an alternate diagnosis, ultimately shown pathologically to be CJD [51].

Management

At present, the etiology and pathogenesis of CBD are unknown. In the future, treatments designed to interfere with the various processes underlying the pathological aggregation of phosphorylated 4R-tau may effectively slow the inexorable progression of the disease. It is likely that breakthroughs in the basic treatment of any of the related tauopathies (e.g. PSP and FTDP-17 owing to tau mutations) will have an impact on the management of CBD. Until then, treatment of CBD is limited to symptomatic interventions and attempts to improve function, concluding with palliative care.

Pharmacological therapies

All treatments suggested to provide some benefit in CBS and CBD are based on open-label anecdotal reports, usually involving small numbers of clinically diagnosed patients and relying exclusively on subjective reports of response.

Parkinsonism

The parkinsonism in CBS is typically unresponsive to levodopa therapy, although transient mild to modest improvements have been reported [4,61,64], including in one of four pathologically confirmed patients [56]. No reported patients with CBS have had a sustained response to levodopa or other dopaminergic therapies [130]. A single report describes levodopa-induced dyskinesia after 18 months of levodopa therapy (800 mg/day) in a patient with confirmed CBD, with decreased dyskinesia but worsening parkinsonism following dose reduction [131]. A small percentage of patients with CBS have reported worsening of motor symptoms with levodopa [61]. While levodopa is the most common anti-parkinsonism medication used, dopamine agonists, selegiline and amantadine, have also been tried, typically with minimal benefit [61,64]. There are limited reports of improvement in parkinsonism with benzodiazepines, anticholinergic medications, baclofen, anticonvulsants, and propranolol [61].

Dystonia

Occasional improvements in dystonia with levodopa, benzodiazepines, anticholinergic drugs, and baclofen have been reported in CBS [61]. Individuals treated with baclofen, dantrolene, and diazepam in a separate series showed no benefit [4]. Targeted botulinum toxin injections may be the most useful intervention, with the majority of patients receiving it describing some improvement [61,64,132]. Three patients with a clenched fist owing to CBS experienced significant improvement in pain and muscle relaxation after botulinum toxin injections targeting the lumbrical and finger flexor muscles, although function remained unchanged [132].

Myoclonus

Benzodiazepines, particularly clonazepam, have been used in patients with myoclonus in CBS to some effect [4,61,64]. Although no improvements with valproic acid, piracetam, or diazepam were obtained in one series [4], trials of valproic acid, gabapentin, levetiracetam, piracetam, and felbamate have been recommended [133]. Levetiracetam 1000 mg/day partially decreased myoclonic and involuntary movements in one recent case report [23].

Tremor

Anticonvulsant medication and propranolol targeting tremor are beneficial only occasionally [61]. Other considerations include benzodiazepines, anticholinergic drugs, levodopa, primidone, and nadolol [133].

Neuropsychiatric and cognitive features

There have been no formal studies of pharmacological therapy for the psychiatric and cognitive aspects of CBS. It may be reasonable to target memory or executive impairment with

acetylcholinesterase inhibitors (AChEI), N-methyl d-aspartate (NMDA) receptor antagonists (e.g. memantine), or dopaminergic agents [133]. While one series found that only 1 of
the 16 CBS patients treated with antidepressant medication reported clinical improvement
[61], Boeve *et al.* report that selective serotonin re-uptake inhibitors (SSRIs) are effective
at both minimizing depression and controlling problematic obsessive-compulsive behaviors [133]. Abulia may respond to AChEI, psychostimulants, and activating antidepressants
[133] and neuroleptics may be useful in patients with dyscontrol [61,133].

Physical therapy and speech therapy

Physical and ancillary therapies in patients with CBS are rarely reported. The profound
apraxia in CBS may reduce responses to physical therapy known to help other disorders
with parkinsonism. Often it greatly limits the patient's ability to learn new strategies when
attempting to improve physical disabilities. Constraint-induced movement therapy, now
used with increasing frequency in stroke patients, was reported to provide benefit for over
two years in one CBS patient, with variable results in others [133]. Long-term locomotor
training has also been reported to benefit a patient with mixed CBS and PSP features [134].
The potential benefits of speech therapy for CBD-related aphasia and speech apraxia are
unknown.

Surgery

While formal studies are lacking, surgery is unlikely to help patients with CBD, as with
most other atypical parkinsonism syndromes. One patient with severe myoclonus and
painful dystonia showed no improvement with stereotactic thalamotomy and right dorsal
rhizotomy of the fifth cervical to first thoracic spinal nerves [4]. In a series of referrals for
failure of deep brain stimulation (DBS), five were related to misdiagnosis, including one
patient with CBS mistaken for essential tremor [135]. There are a number of patients who
have received DBS of the subthalamic nucleus or globus pallidus internus without benefit
(unpublished data).

Palliative therapy

Given the relentless progression of CBS, palliative interventions are an important aspect of
continuing care. Physical supports such as wheelchairs are often required, particularly when
postural instability is prominent. When dysphagia is present, percutaneous endoscopic gastrostomy tube placement must be discussed, although this cannot fully alleviate the risk of
aspiration. Family and caregiver support is critical [130]. In the late stages, palliative and
hospice programs may be appropriate where available.

Conclusion and future directions

Given the broadly based multisystem nature of CBD, it is unlikely that highly effective symptomatic treatments will be developed. Given this and the relentless progression of the disease, the research emphasis needs to focus on understanding the pathogenesis of CBD and
developing neuroprotective or disease-modifying strategies. Understanding the pathological
causes of CBS and CBD and developing potential treatments are closely linked. Better methods of distinguishing the various pathological causes of CBS are clearly needed. Such efforts
are academic, however, unless effective disease-modifying therapies are found.

The two most common general categories of neurodegenerative disease associated with the CBS phenotype are tauopathies and TDP-43 proteinopathies. Treatments directed at altering the pathogenesis of disease will likely differ between these two groups, although treatments may be effective for several different disorders with each sub-category (e.g. CBD, PSP, FTDP-17 owing to tau mutation).

As for all neurodegenerative diseases, multiple pathogenic mechanisms have been proposed in the tauopathies, including mitochondrial dysfunction, oxidative stress, abnormal axonal transport, inflammation, and particularly disturbances in tau metabolism. Putative disease-modifying therapies could be proposed in all of these categories. With respect to tau metabolism, it is known that hyperphosphorylation of tau is a characteristic feature of the tauopathies. Proposed therapeutic targets include decreasing kinase activity or increasing phosphatase activity. The former approach is probably more within the realm of possibility, with two glycogen synthase kinase 3-β (GSK-3β) inhibitors available for clinical use: lithium and valproic acid. Indeed, lithium has been demonstrated to ameliorate disease progression in transgenic mouse models of tauopathy [136] and currently there is a Phase II study of the safety and tolerability of lithium combining patients with CBS and PSP. Alternatively, CBS could be combined with FTD presenting with PNFA (more predictive of underlying CBD pathology). This approach is being used to study the effects of NAPVSIPQ [137], a neuroprotective peptide that stimulates microtubule assembly and reduces tau phosphorylation (A. Boxer, personal communication). The lumping approach recognizes that, although CBS may be a result of a variety of pathologies, the majority of such patients have an underlying tauopathy (particularly if patients with a familial disorder are excluded, removing patients with PGRN mutations). Until more effective biomarkers are available, such lumping together of conditions can be justified in order to encourage advances in the treatment of this otherwise untreatable disorder.

References

1. Rebeiz JJ, Kolodny EH, Richardson EP Jr. Corticodentatonigral degeneration with neuronal achromasia. *Arch Neurol* 1968; **18**: 20–33.

2. Case records of the Massachusetts General Hospital. Weekly clinicopathological exercises. Case 38–1985: a 66-year-old man with progressive neurologic deterioration. *N Engl J Med* 1985; **313**: 739–48.

3. Watts RL, Williams RS, Growdon JD, et al. Corticobasal ganglionic degeneration. *Neurology* 1985; **35** (Suppl 1): 178.

4. Riley DE, Lang AE, Lewis A, et al. Cortical-basal ganglionic degeneration. *Neurology* 1990; **40**: 1203–12.

5. Gibb WR, Luthert PJ, Marsden CD. Corticobasal degeneration. *Brain* 1989; **112**: 1171–92.

6. Doran M, du Plessis DG, Enevoldson TP, et al. Pathological heterogeneity of clinically diagnosed corticobasal degeneration. *J Neurol Sci* 2003; **216**: 127–34.

7. Dickson DW, Bergeron C, Chin SS, et al. Office of Rare Diseases neuropathologic criteria for corticobasal degeneration. *J Neuropathol Exp Neurol* 2002; **61**: 935–46.

8. Hughes AJ, Daniel SE, Ben Shlomo Y, et al. The accuracy of diagnosis of parkinsonian syndromes in a specialist movement disorder service. *Brain* 2002; **125**: 861–70.

9. Togasaki DM, Tanner CM. Epidemiologic aspects. *Adv Neurol* 2000; **82**: 53–9.

10. Schneider JA, Watts RL, Gearing M, et al. Corticobasal degeneration: neuropathologic and clinical heterogeneity. *Neurology* 1997; **48**: 959–69.

11. Katsuse O, Iseki E, Arai T, et al. 4-repeat tauopathy sharing pathological and biochemical features of corticobasal degeneration and progressive supranuclear palsy. *Acta Neuropathol* 2003; **106**: 251–60.

12. Lladó A, Sánchez-Valle R, Rey MJ, et al. Clinicopathological and genetic correlates

of frontotemporal lobar degeneration and corticobasal degeneration. *J Neurol* 2008; **255**: 488–94.

13. López de Munain A, Alzualde A, Gorostidi A, et al. Mutations in progranulin gene: clinical, pathological, and ribonucleic acid expression findings. *Biol Psychiatry* 2008; **63**: 946–52.

14. Keith-Rokosh J, Ang LC. Progressive supranuclear palsy: a review of co-existing neurodegeneration. *Can J Neurol Sci* 2008; **35**: 602–8.

15. Yoshida M. Cellular tau pathology and immunohistochemical study of tau isoforms in sporadic tauopathies. *Neuropathology* 2006; **26**: 457–70.

16. Liu F, Gong CX. Tau exon 10 alternative splicing and tauopathies. *Mol Neurodegener* 2008; **3**: 8.

17. Dickson DW, Litvan I. Corticobasal degeneration. In: Dickson D, ed. *Neurodegeneration: The Molecular Pathology of Dementia and Movement Disorders.* Basel: Neuropath Press, 2003; 115–23.

18. Uryu K, Nakashima-Yasuda H, Forman MS, et al. Concomitant TAR-DNA-binding protein 43 pathology is present in Alzheimer disease and corticobasal degeneration but not in other tauopathies. *J Neuropathol Exp Neurol* 2008; **67**: 555–64.

19. Mirra SS, Murrell JR, Gearing M, et al. Tau pathology in a family with dementia and a P301L mutation in tau. *J Neuropathol Exp Neurol* 1999; **58**: 335–45.

20. Spillantini MG, Yoshida H, Rizzini C, et al. A novel tau mutation (N296N) in familial dementia with swollen achromatic neurons and corticobasal inclusion bodies. *Ann Neurol* 2000; **48**: 939–43.

21. Brown J, Lantos PL, Roques P, et al. Familial dementia with swollen achromatic neurons and corticobasal inclusion bodies: a clinical and pathological study. *J Neurol Sci* 1996; **135**: 21–30.

22. Bugiani O, Murrell JR, Giaccone G, et al. Frontotemporal dementia and corticobasal degeneration in a family with a P301S mutation in tau. *J Neuropathol Exp Neurol* 1999; **58**: 667–77.

23. Rossi G, Marelli C, Farina L, et al. The G389R mutation in the MAPT gene presenting as sporadic corticobasal syndrome. *Mov Disord* 2008; **23**: 892–5.

24. Uchihara T, Nakayama H. Familial tauopathy mimicking corticobasal degeneration an autopsy study on three siblings. *J Neurol Sci* 2006; **246**: 45–51.

25. Tuite PJ, Clark HB, Bergeron C, et al. Clinical and pathologic evidence of corticobasal degeneration and progressive supranuclear palsy in familial tauopathy. *Arch Neurol* 2005; **62**: 1453–7.

26. Houlden H, Baker M, Morris HR, et al. Corticobasal degeneration and progressive supranuclear palsy share a common tau haplotype. *Neurology* 2001; **56**: 1702–6.

27. Webb A, Miller B, Bonasera S, et al. Role of the tau gene region chromosome inversion in progressive supranuclear palsy, corticobasal degeneration, and related disorders. *Arch Neurol* 2008; **65**: 1473–8.

28. Benussi L, Binetti G, Sina E, et al. A novel deletion in progranulin gene is associated with FTDP-17 and CBS. *Neurobiol Aging* 2008; **29**: 427–35.

29. Le Ber I, Camuzat A, Hannequin D, et al. Phenotype variability in progranulin mutation carriers: a clinical, neuropsychological, imaging and genetic study. *Brain* 2008; **131**: 732–46.

30. Gass J, Cannon A, Mackenzie IR, et al. Mutations in progranulin are a major cause of ubiquitin-positive frontotemporal lobar degeneration. *Hum Mol Genet* 2006; **15**: 2988–3001.

31. Masellis M, Momeni P, Meschino W, et al. Novel splicing mutation in the progranulin gene causing familial corticobasal syndrome. *Brain* 2006; **129**: 3115–23.

32. Spina S, Murrell JR, Huey ED, et al. Corticobasal syndrome associated with the A9D Progranulin mutation. *J Neuropathol Exp Neurol* 2007; **66**: 892–900.

33. Baba Y, Uitti RJ, Farrer MJ, et al. Sporadic SCA8 mutation resembling corticobasal degeneration. *Parkinsonism Relat Disord* 2005; **11**: 147–50.

34. Mallucci GR, Campbell TA, Dickinson A, et al. Inherited prion disease with an alanine to valine mutation at codon 117 in the prion protein gene. *Brain* 1999; **122**: 1823–37.

35. Di Maria E, Tabaton M, Vigo T, et al. Corticobasal degeneration shares a common genetic background with progressive supranuclear palsy. *Ann Neurol* 2000; **47**: 374–7.

36. Morris HR, Janssen JC, Bandmann O, et al. The tau gene A0 polymorphism in progressive supranuclear palsy and related neurodegenerative diseases. *J Neurol Neurosurg Psychiatry* 1999; **66**: 665–7.

37. Frank S, Clavaguera F, Tolnay M. Tauopathy models and human neuropathology: similarities and differences. *Acta Neuropathol* 2008; **115**: 39–53.

38. Forman MS, Lal D, Zhang B, et al. Transgenic mouse model of tau pathology in astrocytes leading to nervous system degeneration. *J Neurosci* 2005; **25**: 3539–50.

39. Götz J, Tolnay M, Barmettler R, et al. Oligodendroglial tau filament formation in transgenic mice expressing G272V tau. *Eur J Neurosci* 2001; **13**: 2131–40.

40. Higuchi M, Ishihara T, Zhang B, et al. Transgenic mouse model of tauopathies with glial pathology and nervous system degeneration. *Neuron* 2002; **35**: 433–46.

41. Rinne JO, Lee MS, Thompson PD, et al. Corticobasal degeneration. A clinical study of 36 cases. *Brain* 1994; **117**: 1183–96.

42. Case Records of the Massachusetts General Hospital. Weekly clinicopathological exercises. Case 46–1993: a 75-year-old man with right-sided rigidity, dysarthria, and abnormal gait. *N Engl J Med* 1993; **329**:1560–7.

43. Bhatia KP, Lee MS, Rinne JO, et al. Corticobasal degeneration look-alikes. *Adv Neurol* 2000; **82**: 169–82.

44. Boeve BF, Maraganore DM, Parisi JE, et al. Pathologic heterogeneity in clinically diagnosed corticobasal degeneration. *Neurology* 1999; **53**: 795–800.

45. Josephs KA, Petersen RC, Knopman DS, et al. Clinicopathologic analysis of frontotemporal and corticobasal degenerations and PSP. *Neurology* 2006; **66**: 41–8.

46. Maraganore DM, Boeve B, Parisi J. Disorders mimicking the "classical" clinical syndrome of cortical-basal ganglionic degeneration. *Mov Disord* 1996; **11**: 347.

47. Lang AE, Bergeron C, Pollanen MS, et al. Parietal Pick's disease mimicking cortical-basal ganglionic degeneration. *Neurology* 1994; **44**: 1436–40.

48. Ball JA, Lantos PL, Jackson M, et al. Alien hand sign in association with Alzheimer's histopathology. *J Neurol Neurosurg Psychiatry* 1993; **56**: 1020–3.

49. Wojcieszek J, Lang AE, Jankovic J, et al. Case 1, 1994: what is it? Rapidly progressive aphasia, apraxia, dementia, myoclonus, and parkinsonism. *Mov Disord* 1994; **9**: 358–66.

50. Grimes DA, Bergeron CB, Lang AE. Motor neuron disease-inclusion dementia presenting as cortical-basal ganglionic degeneration. *Mov Disord* 1999; **14**: 674–80.

51. Avanzino L, Marinelli L, Buccolieri A, et al. Creutzfeldt-Jakob disease presenting as corticobasal degeneration: a neurophysiological study. *Neurol Sci* 2006; **27**: 118–21.

52. Kleiner-Fisman G, Bergeron C, Lang AE. Presentation of Creutzfeldt-Jakob disease as acute corticobasal degeneration syndrome. *Mov Disord* 2004; **19**: 948–9.

53. Anschel DJ, Simon DK, Llinas R, et al. Spongiform encephalopathy mimicking corticobasal degeneration. *Mov Disord* 2002; **17**: 606–7.

54. Josephs KA, Dickson DW. Diagnostic accuracy of progressive supranuclear palsy in the Society for Progressive Supranuclear Palsy brain bank. *Mov Disord* 2003; **18**: 1018–26.

55. Osaki Y, Ben Shlomo Y, Lees AJ, et al. Accuracy of clinical diagnosis of progressive supranuclear palsy. *Mov Disord* 2004; **19**: 181–9.

56. Wenning GK, Litvan I, Jankovic J, et al. Natural history and survival of 14 patients with corticobasal degeneration confirmed at postmortem examination. *J Neurol Neurosurg Psychiatry* 1998; **64**: 184–9.

57. Vanvoorst WA, Greenaway MC, Boeve BF, et al. Neuropsychological findings in clinically atypical autopsy confirmed corticobasal degeneration and progressive supranuclear palsy. *Parkinsonism Relat Disord* 2008; **14**: 376–8.

58. Mathuranath PS, Xuereb JH, Bak T, et al. Corticobasal ganglionic degeneration and/or frontotemporal dementia? A report of two overlap cases and review of literature. *J Neurol Neurosurg Psychiatry* 2000; **68**: 304–12.

59. Grimes DA, Lang AE, Bergeron CB. Dementia as the most common presentation of cortical-basal ganglionic

degeneration. *Neurology* 1999;
53: 1969–74.

60. Hasselblatt M, Föllinger S, Steinbach P, et al. Corticobasal degeneration presenting with progressive spasticity. *Neurology* 2007; **68**: 791–2.

61. Kompoliti K, Goetz CG, Boeve BF, et al. Clinical presentation and pharmacological therapy in corticobasal degeneration. *Arch Neurol* 1998; **55**: 957–61.

62. Boeve BF, Lang AE, Litvan I. Corticobasal degeneration and its relationship to progressive supranuclear palsy and frontotemporal dementia. *Ann Neurol* 2003; **54** (Suppl 5): S15–19.

63. Kumar R, Bergeron C, Pollanen M, et al. Cortical-basal Ganglionic Degeneration. In: Jankovic J, Tolosa E, eds. *Parkinson's Disease and Movement Disorders*. Baltimore: Williams and Wilkins, 1998; 297–316.

64. Vanek Z, Jankovic J. Dystonia in corticobasal degeneration. *Mov Disord* 2001; **16**: 252–7.

65. Thompson PD, Day BL, Rothwell JC, et al. The myoclonus in corticobasal degeneration. Evidence for two forms of cortical reflex myoclonus. *Brain* 1994; **117**: 1197–207.

66. Defebvre L. Myoclonus and extrapyramidal diseases. *Neurophysiol Clin* 2006; **36**: 319–25.

67. Leiguarda R, Lees AJ, Merello M, et al. The nature of apraxia in corticobasal degeneration. *J Neurol Neurosurg Psychiatry* 1994; **57**: 455–9.

68. Soliveri P, Piacentini S, Girotti F. Limb apraxia in corticobasal degeneration and progressive supranuclear palsy. *Neurology* 2005; **64**: 448–53.

69. Scepkowski LA, Cronin-Golomb A. The alien hand: cases, categorizations, and anatomical correlates. *Behav Cogn Neurosci Rev* 2003; **2**: 261–77.

70. Bergeron C, Pollanen MS, Weyer L, et al. Unusual clinical presentations of cortical-basal ganglionic degeneration. *Ann Neurol* 1996; **40**: 893–900.

71. Fitzgerald DB, Drago V, Jeong Y, et al. Asymmetrical alien hands in corticobasal degeneration. *Mov Disord* 2007; **22**: 581–4.

72. Pillon B, Blin J, Vidailhet M, et al. The neuropsychological pattern of corticobasal degeneration: comparison with progressive supranuclear palsy and Alzheimer's disease. *Neurology* 1995; **45**: 1477–83.

73. Graham NL, Bak TH, Hodges JR. Corticobasal degeneration as a cognitive disorder. *Mov Disord* 2003; **18**: 1224–32.

74. Halpern C, McMillan C, Moore P, et al. Calculation impairment in neurodegenerative diseases. *J Neurol Sci* 2003; **208**: 31–8.

75. Frattali CM, Grafman J, Patronas N, et al. Language disturbances in corticobasal degeneration. *Neurology* 2000; **54**: 990–2.

76. Graham NL, Bak T, Patterson K, et al. Language function and dysfunction in corticobasal degeneration. *Neurology* 2003; **61**: 493–9.

77. Vidailhet M, Rivaud-Péchoux S. Eye movement disorders in corticobasal degeneration. *Adv Neurol* 2000; **82**: 161–7.

78. Garbutt S, Matlin A, Hellmuth J, et al. Oculomotor function in frontotemporal lobar degeneration, related disorders and Alzheimer's disease. *Brain* 2008; **131**: 1268–81.

79. Mendez MF. Corticobasal ganglionic degeneration with Balint's syndrome. *J Neuropsychiatry Clin Neurosci* 2000; **12**: 273–5.

80. Okuda B, Kodama N, Tachibana H, et al. Visuomotor ataxia in corticobasal degeneration. *Mov Disord* 2000; **15**: 337–40.

81. Nagaoka K, Ookawa S, Maeda K. A case of corticobasal degeneration presenting with visual hallucination. *Rinsho Shinkeigaku* 2004; **44**: 193–7.

82. Pardini M, Huey ED, Cavanagh AL, et al. Olfactory function in corticobasal syndrome and frontotemporal dementia. *Arch Neurol* 2009; **66**: 92–6.

83. Litvan I, Cummings JL, Mega M. Neuropsychiatric features of corticobasal degeneration. *J Neurol Neurosurg Psychiatry* 1998; **65**: 717–21.

84. Thumler BH, Urban PP, Davids E, et al. Dysarthria and pathological laughter/crying as presenting symptoms of corticobasal-ganglionic degeneration syndrome. *J Neurol* 2003; **250**: 1107–8.

85. Kertesz A, Martinez-Lage P, Davidson W, et al. The corticobasal degeneration syndrome overlaps progressive aphasia and frontotemporal dementia. *Neurology* 2000; **55**: 1368–75.

86. Kertesz A, Munoz DG. Diagnostic controversies: is CBD part of the "pick complex"? *Adv Neurol* 2000; **82**: 223–31.

87. Kertesz A, McMonagle P, Blair M, et al. The evolution and pathology of frontotemporal dementia. *Brain* 2005; **128**: 1996–2005.

88. McMonagle P, Blair M, Kertesz A. Corticobasal degeneration and progressive aphasia. *Neurology* 2006; **67**: 1444–51.

89. Hodges JR, Davies RR, Xuereb JH, et al. Clinicopathological correlates in frontotemporal dementia. *Ann Neurol* 2004; **56**: 399–406.

90. Murray R, Neumann M, Forman MS, et al. Cognitive and motor assessment in autopsy-proven corticobasal degeneration. *Neurology* 2007; **68**: 1274–83.

91. Josephs KA, Duffy JR, Strand EA, et al. Clinicopathological and imaging correlates of progressive aphasia and apraxia of speech. *Brain* 2006; **129**: 1385–98.

92. Josephs KA, Duffy JR. Apraxia of speech and nonfluent aphasia: a new clinical marker for corticobasal degeneration and progressive supranuclear palsy. *Curr Opin Neurol* 2008; **21**: 688–92.

93. Litvan I, Grimes DA, Lang AE, et al. Clinical features differentiating patients with postmortem confirmed progressive supranuclear palsy and corticobasal degeneration. *J Neurol* 1999; **246**(Suppl 2): II1–5.

94. Tang-Wai DF, Josephs KA, Boeve BF, et al. Pathologically confirmed corticobasal degeneration presenting with visuospatial dysfunction. *Neurology* 2003; **61**: 1134–5.

95. DePold Hohler A, Ransom BR, Chun MR, et al. The youngest reported case of corticobasal degeneration. *Parkinsonism Relat Disord* 2003; **10**: 47–50.

96. Borroni B, Malinverno M, Gardoni F, et al. Tau forms in CSF as a reliable biomarker for progressive supranuclear palsy. *Neurology* 2008; **71**: 1796–803.

97. Arai H, Morikawa Y, Higuchi M, et al. Cerebrospinal fluid tau levels in neurodegenerative diseases with distinct tau-related pathology. *Biochem Biophys Res Commun* 1997; **236**: 262–4.

98. Urakami K, Mori M, Wada K, et al. A comparison of tau protein in cerebrospinal fluid between corticobasal degeneration and progressive supranuclear palsy. *Neurosci Lett* 1999; **259**: 127–9.

99. Urakami K, Wada K, Arai H, et al. Diagnostic significance of tau protein in cerebrospinal fluid from patients with corticobasal degeneration or progressive supranuclear palsy. *J Neurol Sci* 2001; **183**: 95–8.

100. Mitani K, Furiya Y, Uchihara T, et al. Increased total CSF tau protein in corticobasal degeneration has also been reported in patients with CBGD compared to normal controls. *J Neurol* 1998; **245**: 44–6.

101. Yasui K, Inoue Y, Kanbayashi T, et al. CSF orexin levels of Parkinson's disease, dementia with Lewy bodies, progressive supranuclear palsy and corticobasal degeneration. *J Neurol Sci* 2006; **250**: 120–3.

102. Noguchi M, Yoshita M, Matsumoto Y, et al. Decreased beta-amyloid peptide 42 in cerebrospinal fluid of patients with progressive supranuclear palsy and corticobasal degeneration. *J Neurol Sci* 2005; **237**: 61–5.

103. Brettschneider J, Petzold A, Sussmuth SD, et al. Neurofilament heavy-chain NfH(SMI35) in cerebrospinal fluid supports the differential diagnosis of Parkinsonian syndromes. *Mov Disord* 2006; **21**: 2224–7.

104. Kanemaru K, Mitani K, Yamanouchi H. Cerebrospinal fluid homovanillic acid levels are not reduced in early corticobasal degeneration. *Neurosci Lett* 1998; **245**: 121–2.

105. Belfor N, Amici S, Boxer AL, et al. Clinical and neuropsychological features of corticobasal degeneration. *Mech Ageing Dev* 2006; **127**: 203–7.

106. Warren JD, Mummery CJ, Al-Din AS, et al. Corticobasal degeneration syndrome with basal ganglia calcification: Fahr's disease as a corticobasal look-alike? *Mov Disord* 2002; **17**: 563–7.

107. Mridula KR, Alladi S, Varma DR, et al. Corticobasal syndrome due to a thalamic tuberculoma and focal cortical atrophy. *J Neurol Neurosurg Psychiatry* 2008; **79**: 107–8.

108. Koyama M, Yagishita A, Nakata Y, et al. Imaging of corticobasal degeneration syndrome. *Neuroradiology* 2007; **49**: 905–12.

109. Ukmar M, Moretti R, Torre P, et al. Corticobasal degeneration: structural

and functional MRI and single-photon emission computed tomography. *Neuroradiology* 2003; **45**: 708–12.

110. Boxer AL, Geschwind MD, Belfor N, et al. Patterns of brain atrophy that differentiate corticobasal degeneration syndrome from progressive supranuclear palsy. *Arch Neurol* 2006; **63**: 81–6.

111. Josephs KA, Tang-Wai DF, Edland SD, et al. Correlation between antemortem magnetic resonance imaging findings and pathologically confirmed corticobasal degeneration. *Arch Neurol* 2004; **61**: 1881–4.

112. Josephs KA, Whitwell JL, Dickson DW, et al. Voxel-based morphometry in autopsy proven PSP and CBD. *Neurobiol Aging* 2008; **29**: 280–9.

113. Gröschel K, Hauser TK, Luft A, et al. Magnetic resonance imaging-based volumetry differentiates progressive supranuclear palsy from corticobasal degeneration. *Neuroimage* 2004; **21**: 714–24.

114. Vion-Dury J, Rochefort N, Michotey P, et al. Proton magnetic resonance neurospectroscopy and EEG cartography in corticobasal degeneration: correlations with neuropsychological signs. *J Neurol Neurosurg Psychiatry* 2004; **75**: 1352–5.

115. Coulier IM, de Vries JJ, Leenders KL. Is FDG-PET a useful tool in clinical practice for diagnosing corticobasal ganglionic degeneration? *Mov Disord* 2003; **18**: 1175–8.

116. Laureys S, Salmon E, Garraux G, et al. Fluorodopa uptake and glucose metabolism in early stages of corticobasal degeneration. *J Neurol* 1999; **246**: 1151–8.

117. Eckert T, Barnes A, Dhawan V, et al. FDG PET in the differential diagnosis of parkinsonian disorders. *Neuroimage* 2005; **26**: 912–21.

118. Klaffke S, Kuhn AA, Plotkin M, et al. Dopamine transporters, D2 receptors, and glucose metabolism in corticobasal degeneration. *Mov Disord* 2006; **21**: 1724–7.

119. Nagasawa H, Tanji H, Nomura H, et al. PET study of cerebral glucose metabolism and fluorodopa uptake in patients with corticobasal degeneration. *J Neurol Sci* 1996; **139**: 210–7.

120. Gerhard A, Watts J, Trender-Gerhard I, et al. In vivo imaging of microglial activation with [11C](R)-PK 11195 PET in corticobasal degeneration. *Mov Disord* 2004; **19**: 1221–6.

121. Sawle GV, Brooks DJ, Marsden CD, et al. Corticobasal degeneration. A unique pattern of regional cortical oxygen hypometabolism and striatal fluorodopa uptake demonstrated by positron emission tomography. *Brain* 1991; **114**: 541–56.

122. Walter U, Dressler D, Wolters A, et al. Sonographic discrimination of corticobasal degeneration vs progressive supranuclear palsy. *Neurology* 2004; **63**: 504–9.

123. Tashiro K, Ogata K, Goto Y, et al. EEG findings in early-stage corticobasal degeneration and progressive supranuclear palsy: a retrospective study and literature review. *Clin Neurophysiol* 2006; **117**: 2236–42.

124. Chen R, Ashby P, Lang AE. Stimulus-sensitive myoclonus in akinetic-rigid syndromes. *Brain* 1992; **115**: 1875–88.

125. Monza D, Ciano C, Scaioli V, et al. Neurophysiological features in relation to clinical signs in clinically diagnosed corticobasal degeneration. *Neurol Sci* 2003; **24**: 16–23.

126. Brunt ER, van Weerden TW, Pruim J, et al. Unique myoclonic pattern in corticobasal degeneration. *Mov Disord* 1995; **10**: 132–42.

127. Grosse P, Kühn A, Cordivari C, et al. Coherence analysis in the myoclonus of corticobasal degeneration. *Mov Disord* 2003; **18**: 1345–50.

128. Trompetto C, Buccolieri A, Marchese R, et al. Impairment of transcallosal inhibition in patients with corticobasal degeneration. *Clin Neurophysiol* 2003; **114**: 2181–7.

129. Wolters A, Classen J, Kunesch E, et al. Measurements of transcallosally mediated cortical inhibition for differentiating parkinsonian syndromes. *Mov Disord* 2004; **19**: 518–28.

130. Lang AE. Treatment of progressive supranuclear palsy and corticobasal degeneration. *Mov Disord* 2005; **20** (Suppl 12): S83–91.

131. Frucht S, Fahn S, Chin S, et al. Levodopa-induced dyskinesias in autopsy-proven cortical-basal ganglionic degeneration. *Mov Disord* 2000; **15**: 340–3.

132. Cordivari C, Misra VP, Catania S, et al. Treatment of dystonic clenched fist with

botulinum toxin. *Mov Disord* 2001; **16**: 907–13.

133. Boeve BF, Josephs KA, Drubach DA. Current and future management of the corticobasal syndrome and corticobasal degeneration. *Handb Clin Neurol* 2008; **89**: 533–48.

134. Steffen TM, Boeve BF, Mollinger-Riemann LA, et al. Long-term locomotor training for gait and balance in a patient with mixed progressive supranuclear palsy and corticobasal degeneration. *Phys Ther* 2007; **87**: 1078–87.

135. Okun MS, Tagliati M, Pourfar M, et al. Management of referred deep brain stimulation failures: a retrospective analysis from 2 movement disorders centers. *Arch Neurol* 2005; **62**: 1250–5.

136. Noble W, Planel E, Zehr C, et al. Inhibition of glycogen synthase kinase-3 by lithium correlates with reduced tauopathy and degeneration in vivo. *Proc Natl Acad Sci USA* 2005; **102**: 6990–5.

137. Matsuoka Y, Jouroukhin Y, Gray AJ, et al. A neuronal microtubule-interacting agent, NAPVSIPQ, reduces tau pathology and enhances cognitive function in a mouse model of Alzheimer's disease. *J Pharmacol Exp Ther* 2008; **325**: 146–53.

Parkinsonism – other causes

David E. Riley

The majority of patients with parkinsonism have Parkinson's disease (PD), or disorders covered in other chapters of this book. However, many other patients do not fall readily into these diagnostic categories. In such cases, consideration should be given to other etiologies, particularly as early recognition of some disorders can lead to reversal of deficits or, at least, alteration of the progression of disability. In some cases, intervention can ultimately prevent death.

The syndrome of parkinsonism has an ever-growing number of causes, to a point where listing them has become somewhat unwieldy. In this chapter, while a comprehensive differential diagnosis of parkinsonism is provided in the tables, an attempt is made to provide guidance with practical value by highlighting the most important disorders according to frequency and treatability.

Drug-induced parkinsonism

With the introduction of dopamine receptor-blocking drugs for schizophrenia in the 1950s, drugs rapidly became the second most common cause of parkinsonism [1]. Approximately 20% of patients on long-term antipsychotic therapy develop drug-induced parkinsonism (DIP) [2]. Genetic predisposition may underlie much of an individual's susceptibility [3]. Other risk factors for DIP include increasing age, female gender, and poor performance on cognitive testing [4,5]. DIP probably mimics PD more closely than any other form of parkinsonism, often including a resting tremor. One possible reason for this resemblance is that antidopaminergic drugs may unmask actual PD [6,7], rather than simply reproducing its dopamine deprivation. Aside from the history of a potentially causative medication, supportive clinical features, when present, include the relatively rapid onset and symmetrical presentation [8]. DIP may also be differentiated from PD by olfactory testing, cardiac scintigraphy, and dopamine transporter brain imaging [9,10].

All antipsychotic agents may cause DIP [11], with the exception of clozapine, while DIP as a result of quetiapine is distinctly rare [12–15]. Dopamine receptor blockers used to treat gastrointestinal complaints, such as metoclopramide, prochlorperazine, and levosulpiride [16], and vertigo, such as thiethylperazine [17], or menopausal symptoms, such as veralipride [18], are frequently culpable [7] and are underappreciated as causes of parkinsonism [19]. It may be necessary to question patients (and caregivers) regarding problems for which they have been treated to jar an appropriate memory, rather than simply requesting an unselected list of medications. In addition to these medications, a large catalogue of drugs

Handbook of Atypical Parkinsonism, eds. Carlo Colosimo, David E. Riley, and Gregor K. Wenning. Published by Cambridge University Press. © Cambridge University Press 2011.

has caused parkinsonism on an idiosyncratic basis (Table 6.1) [20]. Parkinsonism induced by the calcium channel blockers cinnarizine and flunarizine is common in countries where those drugs are available [21].

The prognosis of DIP is highly favorable, provided patients are able to discontinue the offending drug. Complete resolution of symptoms and signs may take more than one year, in the case of dopamine receptor blockers.

Table 6.1 Drugs reported to induce parkinsonism

Alphamethyldopa [151]
Amiodarone [152]
Amoxapine [153]
Amphotericin B [154]
Aprindine [155]
Bethanechol (intraventricular) [156]
Budesonide [157]
Buphormine [155]
Bupropion [158]
Calcium-channel blockers [159] (amlodipine [160], cinnarizine, flunarizine [21,161], diltiazem [162], verapamil [163])
Captopril [164]
Catecholamine depletors (reserpine [165], tetrabenazine [166])
Cephaloridine [167]
Chloroquine [168]
Cimetidine [169]
Cyclosporine [170]
Cytosine arabinoside [171]
Diazepam [172]
Distigmine bromide [173]
Disulfiram [174,175]
Dopamine receptor blockers (see text)
5-Fluorouracil [176]
Hexamethylmelamine [177]
Interferon-alpha [178]
Levetiracetam [179]
Lithium [180,181]
Meperidine [182]
Methotrexate [183]
Milnacipran [184]
Nizatidine [185]
Octreotide [186]

Table 6.1 (cont.)

Pentoxifylline [187]
Perhexiline [188]
Phenelzine [189]
Phenytoin [190]
Pregabalin [191]
Prenylamine [192]
Procaine [193]
Propiverine [194]
Pyridostigmine [195]
Serotonin-specific reuptake inhibitors (fluoxetine [196], paroxetine [197], sertraline [198])
Thiethylperazine [17]
Trazodone [199]
Trimetazidine [200,201]
Valproate [202]
Veralipride [18]

Toxic causes of parkinsonism

Numerous toxins have been implicated as causes of secondary parkinsonism (Table 6.2). The most notorious toxic cause is likely 1-methyl-4-phenyl-1,2,3,6-tetrahydropyridine (MPTP). This toxin was a byproduct of illicit synthetic meperidine synthesis that produced subacute severe parkinsonism in intravenous drug addicts in California in the 1980s [22]. The MPP$^+$ metabolite of MPTP selectively damages pigmented substantia nigra neurons, possibly through the dopamine transporter system [23]. Although it affected only a small number of individuals, MPTP parkinsonism became famous because it sparked an intensive search for environmental causes of PD [24,25], and because it led to the development of animal models of parkinsonism that remain in frequent use and continue to see new applications [26].

Manganese-induced parkinsonism (MIP) was first described in 1837 [27]. Most cases have occurred in workplace settings where there is exposure to extremely high levels of manganese dust, such as mining and ore processing. Symptoms begin during the exposure period. The clinical presentation consists of a symmetrical akinetic-rigid syndrome with early gait or balance abnormalities, early appearance of dystonia, particularly a cock-walk gait or facial grimacing, relatively rapid progression to disability, and no sustained response to levodopa [28]. T1-weighted MRI may show hyperintensities in the globus pallidus bilaterally during the period of exposure. The majority of patients stabilize after removal from manganese exposure and may improve, although usually only partially, with gait impairment typically being the most vexing residual problem. Pathological studies show degeneration in the globus pallidus, and occasionally the striatum [29]. MIP has become rare as an occupational disorder owing to improvements in industrial safety. However, it has regained prominence, mainly in Eastern Europe, as a hazard of methcathinone abuse [30]. Methcathinone is a stimulant drug often manufactured in home laboratories using a process involving potassium permanganate, the source of the manganese poisoning [31]. Clinical findings and the prognosis in these patients are typical of MIP [32].

Table 6.2 Toxins reported to induce parkinsonism

Betel nut (plus antipsychotics) [203]

Carbon monoxide [204]

Contrast agent for cardiac catheterization [205]

Cyanide [206]

Ethanol intoxication [207], ethanol withdrawal [208]

Ethylene glycol [209]

Herbicides (paraquat [210], diquat [211], glyphosate [212])

Heroin [213]

Hydrogen sulfide [214]

Kava-kava [215]

Manganese [216]

Maneb (manganese ethylene-bis-dithiocarbamate) [210]

Mercury [217]

Methanol [209]

Methcathinone (manganese ephedrone) [30,32]

MPTP (1-methyl-4-phenyl-1,2,3,6-tetrahydropyridine) [218]

Organic solvents (carbon disulfide [219], n-hexane [220], toluene [221], trichloroethylene [222]) [223,224]

Organophosphate insecticide poisoning [225]

Petroleum products [226]

Metabolic disorders causing parkinsonism

Metabolic disorders (Table 6.3) are uncommon causes of parkinsonism. To some degree, this is because of the lack of a direct relationship between parkinsonism and the most common metabolic disorders. While hypothyroidism and PD are often compared [33,34], and may have some clinical similarities (along with depression), there are no reported cases of hypothyroidism causing parkinsonism. Neither is diabetes mellitus known to cause parkinsonism directly, although it is a major risk factor for the vascular type of parkinsonism [35]. Despite their rarity, it is important to be able to recognize some metabolic disorders, particularly Wilson's disease, because early intervention can arrest progression of the condition. Many metabolic disorders are hereditary. Sedel and colleagues proposed that the following features should suggest the occurrence of an inborn error of metabolism: acute to subacute onset in childhood, recessive or X-linked inheritance, a mixture of a movement disorder with other neurological signs, and inability to apply a diagnosis of a classical movement disorder [36].

S.A.K. Wilson described a hereditary form of progressive lenticular degeneration [37] occurring in association with hepatic cirrhosis, a disease that came to bear his name. Wilson's disease (WD) is a truly multisystem disorder with potential hematological, renal, ophthalmic, and other organ involvement. In a majority of patients, the initial hepatic stage (usually occurring during adolescence) is asymptomatic, and the patient goes on to develop neurological and psychiatric complications, typically between the ages of 17 and 25 years and rarely after 40 years old [38]. Neurological presentations are varied, but often revolve

Table 6.3 Metabolic causes of parkinsonism

Aceruloplasminemia [227]
Acquired chronic hepatocerebral degeneration [228]
Acute liver failure [229]
Alexander's disease [230]
Anoxic encephalopathy [231]
Aromatic amino acid decarboxylase deficiency
Central pontine myelinolysis [232]
Cerebrotendinous xanthomatosis [233]
Ceroid lipofuscinosis [234]
Dihydropteridine reductase deficiency [235]
Extrapontine myelinolysis [236]
Fabry's disease [237]
Folate deficiency [238]
Gaucher's disease [239]
GM1 gangliosidosis [240]
GM2 gangliosidosis [241]
Guanosine triphosphate cyclohydrolase 1 (GTPCH1) deficiency (dopa-responsive dystonia) [51]
Heatstroke [242]
Hemodialysis [49]
Hereditary hemochromatosis [50]
Homocystinuria [243]
Mitochondrial respiratory chain disorders [244]
Neurodegeneration with brain iron accumulation type 1 [227]
Neuroferritinopathy [245]
Niemann–Pick type C [141]
Pantothenate kinase-associated neurodegeneration [246]
Phenylketonuria [247]
Polyglucosan body disease [248]
Pyruvate dehydrogenase deficiency [249]
Rapid-onset dystonia-parkinsonism [52]
Total patenteral nutrition [48]
Tyrosine hydroxylase deficiency [250]

around a syndrome that is predominantly parkinsonism, dystonia, or cerebellar tremor and ataxia [39]. The diagnosis of WD hinges on the identification of copper metabolism abnormalities including corneal copper deposits known as Kayser–Fleischer rings, low serum copper and ceruloplasmin levels, high copper excretion in the urine, and high copper levels in liver biopsy samples. Supportive diagnostic evidence may include T2-weighted hyperintensities in the basal ganglia, thalami, brainstem, and cerebral white matter [40].

WD is an autosomal recessive disorder as a result of mutations in *ATP7B*, a gene coding for a transmembrane copper-transporting ATPase on chromosome 13 [41]. Dozens of different mutations are known, and genetic testing is not readily accomplished without whole gene sequencing. WD is uniformly fatal if undetected and untreated. Treatment consists of lifelong copper-chelation therapy initiated with either tetrathiomolybdate or trientine [42], and maintained with either zinc or trientine. Stabilization of the clinical state is typical, and some WD patients experience significant reversal of disease manifestations.

Acquired hepatocerebral degeneration occurs in the setting of non-Wilsonian cirrhosis and presents with a similar variety of clinical manifestations as its congenital or hereditary counterpart, WD, including ataxia, tremor, parkinsonism, dystonia, myoclonus, and chorea [43]. Cognitive and behavioral impairment is also common. Parkinsonism may be the predominant manifestation [44]. Liver disease is usually known and advanced, but may be cryptic. The copper metabolism abnormalities found in WD are lacking. MRI discloses T1-hyperintensity in the putamen and globus pallidus. Clinical and radiological similarities have implicated basal ganglia manganese deposition in the pathogenesis [45]. However, parkinsonism has also been attributed to hyperammonemia in chronic liver failure because of portal vein thrombosis [46]. Conventional treatment for hepatic encephalopathy provides inconsistent symptomatic benefit. Liver transplantation has been curative in anecdotal reports [47]. Manganese intoxication has also been identified as the pathogenetic mechanism for parkinsonism complicating total parenteral nutrition [48] and maintenance hemodialysis [49]. Hereditary hemochromatosis is a known cause of hepatocerebral degeneration. However, recent cases of parkinsonism in patients with hemochromatosis have shown T2-weighted MRI basal ganglia hypointensities, more consistent with abnormal levels of iron accumulation [50]. Response to phlebotomy and anti-parkinsonian medication has been inconsistent.

Guanosine triphosphate cyclohydrolase 1 (GTPCH1) deficiency classically presents as childhood-onset dopa-responsive dystonia. However, affected adults may present with a predominantly parkinsonian syndrome [51]. Rapid-onset dystonia-parkinsonism (RODP) is a rare, unique syndrome the name of which describes its most salient clinical features [52]. It is produced by missense mutations in the *ATP1A3* gene. The parkinsonism of RODP is predominantly akinetic-rigid with little tremor and prominent disequilibrium. A growing number of mitochondrial respiratory chain disorders have been associated with parkinsonism [53–57].

Infection-related parkinsonism

Infectious and post-infectious parkinsonism are historically important. In the early twentieth century, a global epidemic of encephalitis lethargica (EL) led to postencephalitic parkinsonism (PEP), which for decades afterward was the most common type of parkinsonism. In addition to a predominantly akinetic-rigid syndrome, distinctive clinical features included young onset, excess somnolence and other sleep disturbances, oculogyric crises, behavioral changes, dystonia, and tics. Although EL-related PEP showed typical hallmarks of viral infections, the infectious nature of this illness remains an assumption, because no causative agent has been identified. Recent investigations have implicated post-infectious autoimmune mechanisms [58,59]. The original cohort of EL-related PEP has almost all died, and the disorder has occurred only sporadically in recent times [60].

The most common infectious disease setting for parkinsonism currently is HIV infection. In most cases, the parkinsonism is a result of HIV encephalitis [61]. Alternative mechanisms include opportunistic abscesses acting as mass lesions, such as toxoplasma abscesses in the basal ganglia [62] and cryptococcal lesions in the substantia nigra [63], or drug treatment [64,65]. The incidence of HIV-encephalopathy parkinsonism may have declined since the advent of antiretroviral therapy [66], which can produce remissions in individuals already affected [67]. However, it has been argued that HIV infection and retroviral therapy accelerate the aging process and lead to earlier onset of degenerative diseases such as PD [68].

The distinction between infectious and post-infectious parkinsonism is not clear-cut in many instances, either label having been applied in published reports retrospectively, depending on whether and when the parkinsonism resolved. One usually sees one of two scenarios: a transient parkinsonism in the setting of an acute encephalitis, or persistent parkinsonism developing as encephalitis evolves or after the acute infection is resolving (Table 6.4). Japanese and West Nile encephalitides have been associated with both syndromes [69]. In addition to viral encephalitis, post-infectious parkinsonism also has occurred following streptococcal infections [70]. Cysticercosis of the nervous system can cause parkinsonism as a brainstem ependymitis [71], or indirectly through the mechanism of obstructive hydrocephalus [72,73]. A PSP-like syndrome has been attributed to Whipple's disease [74] and to Creutzfeldt–Jakob disease [75].

Table 6.4 Infectious disease and parkinsonism

Aspergillosis/mucormycosis [251]
Creutzfeldt–Jakob disease [252]
Cryptococcosis [63]
Cysticercosis [71]
Encephalitis with persistent parkinsonism (postencephalitic parkinsonism)
Coxsackie virus meningoencephalitis [253,254]
Encephalitis lethargica (see text)
Influenza [255]
Japanese encephalitis [256]
Measles [257]
Mumps [114]
Polio [258]
West Nile meningoencephalitis [69]
Western equine encephalitis [259]
Encephalitis with transient parkinsonism
Epstein–Barr virus encephalitis [260]
Herpes simplex [261]
Japanese encephalitis [262]
St. Louis encephalitis [263]
West Nile meningoencephalitis [69]

Table 6.4 (cont.)

Gerstmann–Sträussler–Scheinker disease [264]

HIV encephalopathy [61,67]

Malaria [265]

Mycoplasma infection [266]

Postvaccinal parkinsonism [212,267,268]

Prion diseases – atypical [269,270]

Progressive multifocal leukoencephalopathy [271]

Subacute sclerosing panencephalitis [272,273]

Syphilis [274]

Toxoplasmosis [62]

Tuberculosis [275,276]

Whipple's disease [277,278]

Structural lesions causing parkinsonism

As the name suggests, this is a category of parkinsonism that is highly dependent on imaging technology for proper diagnosis (Table 6.5). Vascular disease is an important cause of parkinsonism, accounting for 3–6% of all cases [76]. The relationship between parkinsonism and cerebrovascular disease is a complex one, beginning with McDonald Critchley's description of arteriosclerotic parkinsonism in 1929 [77]. Critchley's concept experienced widespread skepticism in subsequent years. However, the advent of modern imaging techniques coupled with greater attention paid to nuances of clinical features of patients with parkinsonism has led to the acceptance of not one but several syndromes of vascular parkinsonism (VP) separate from PD [78]. These can be divided broadly into the focal or unilateral effects of single vascular lesions, and the cumulative effects of multiple or diffuse ischemic events. Patients typically have risk factors associated with vascular disease, mainly hypertension and diabetes mellitus, and there may be a prior history of stroke. VP may also be seen in the context of rarer vascular disorders, such as antiphospholipid syndrome [79], polyarteritis nodosa [80], mixed cryoglobulinemia [81], moyamoya disease [82], and cerebral autosomal dominant arteriopathy with subcortical infarcts and leukoencephalopathy (CADASIL) [83]. Vascular disease may also underlie some cases of progressive supranuclear palsy [84].

The most common vascular syndrome is a gait disorder that has been termed lower-body parkinsonism [85]. It consists of a shuffling gait, often with considerable freezing resembling advanced PD, but with a wider base, more upright posture, and preserved arm swing. There is no tremor and speech, writing, and dexterity are spared or minimally involved. There may be evidence of prior stroke in the form of unilateral weakness, hyperreflexia, a Babinski sign, or other pathological reflexes [86]. Lower-body parkinsonism is associated most often with numerous small, often confluent cerebral white matter infarctions seen on MRI. Unfortunately, there is no general agreement on what proportion of white matter needs to be involved to establish a causal association. Basal ganglia infarcts appear to be less likely to produce this syndrome [87]. Other investigations have yielded mixed results [88], although many investigators find dopamine transporter imaging useful in distinguishing VP from

Table 6.5 Structural lesions causing parkinsonism

Aneurysm of the middle cerebral artery [279]
Basal ganglia angioma, cyst, or tumor [99,280,281]
Calcification of the basal ganglia (see text)
Dural arteriovenous fistula [101]
Gliomatosis cerebri [282,283]
Hemangioblastoma [284]
Hydrocephalus (see text)
Meningioma [285,286]
Midbrain angioma, cyst, hemorrhage, projectile, or tumor [97,287–291]
Pineal region angioma, cyst, or tumor [100,292,293]
Posterior fossa cyst [294]
Subdural hematoma [295,296]
Thalamic angioma, cyst, or tumor [297]
Vascular parkinsonism (see text)

PD [9]. There may be a step-wise or rapid course, but more often the evolution is gradual, reflecting the progressive accumulation of ischemic lesions, none of which is sufficient to cause a clinical disturbance on its own. Levodopa may be beneficial in a minority of patients [85], and this response may be related to the involvement of the nigrostriatal tract by the vascular disease [85,89]. A similar clinical picture occurs with Binswanger's disease [90] or marked dilation of perivascular spaces, known as *état criblé* [91].

A less common presentation of VP consists of focal or unilateral findings suggestive of single vascular lesions [92–94]. A history of an abrupt onset characteristic of ischemic infarction [95], vasculitis [96], primary hemorrhage [97], or venous thrombosis [98] may be present, but is not always elicitable. Conversely, a static or progressive course has been reported in association with vascular mass lesions such as cavernous angiomata in the basal ganglia [99] or pineal region [100], and dural arteriovenous fistulae [101].

Hydrocephalus in both obstructive and non-obstructive varieties may cause parkinsonism. Obstructive hydrocephalus may mimic the full syndrome of PD, and may be levodopa-responsive [102]. Over-drainage after successful shunting can also precipitate parkinsonism [103]. A particular form known as normal pressure hydrocephalus (NPH) produces a combination of dementia, parkinsonian gait, and urinary incontinence. This is a somewhat controversial condition because it is considered overdiagnosed by some and underdiagnosed by others. Differentiation from PD usually is not difficult because of the disproportionate gait disturbance in NPH [104], but the full clinical triad is not always found, and exceptionally there may be diagnostic confusion with PD [105]. The onset is in late adulthood. The etiology is unknown. Ventricular dilation may be difficult to assess in elderly patients with atrophic increase of cerebrospinal fluid (CSF) spaces. In addition to ventriculomegaly, MRI in a majority of NPH patients will show white matter lesions, typically at the poles of the lateral ventricles, that may be reversible [106]. Approximately 75% of patients will experience substantial relief of symptoms from ventriculoperitoneal (VP) shunting [107,108]. A large-volume withdrawal of CSF by lumbar puncture has been recommended [109] to predict responsiveness to VP shunting, which is the definitive therapeutic procedure.

Calcification of the basal ganglia (CBG) usually occurs as a hereditary disorder of unknown pathogenesis or secondary to a disorder of calcium metabolism. The most characteristic diagnostic feature is dense calcium deposition highly visible on CT scans in the striatum, pallidum, and other structures including the thalamus, dentate nuclei, and subcortical white matter. Despite striking imaging abnormalities, approximately one-third of patients have no clinical manifestations [110]. In symptomatic patients, parkinsonism is the most common presentation [111]. Cognitive impairment is common. CBG has also been associated with a PSP-like clinical presentation [112]. In patients in whom a metabolic disorder can be identified, such as hypoparathyroidism, treatment of the underlying disturbance can lead to neurological remission [113]. A case of dystonia, athetosis, and parkinsonism with calcification of the basal ganglia and thalamus followed mumps encephalitis [114].

Degenerative diseases causing parkinsonism

This chapter will consider degenerative disorders (Table 6.6) other than the defined familial syndromes known as PARK diseases [115]. Spinocerebellar degenerations, more commonly known as spinocerebellar ataxias (SCAs), are hereditary disorders producing a combination of cerebellar dysfunction and spasticity in most cases. Autosomal dominant SCAs may include parkinsonism in their clinical repertoire, but usually in addition to the more typical ataxia with or without corticospinal tract symptoms and signs; this clinical picture may suggest a diagnosis of the cerebellar type of multiple system atrophy. Seldom will SCAs present with relatively pure parkinsonism, typical or atypical; such cases have been associated with SCA2 [116,117], SCA3 [118], SCA6 [119], SCA8, and SCA17 [120] mutations. Prevalence surveys among patients with typical and atypical parkinsonism demonstrate that these associations are rare [121–124]. The finding of a SCA mutation does not prove causation of the clinical features [125]. Widespread screening for SCA mutations among patients with parkinsonism is not indicated at present.

Parkinsonism is associated with the early onset of Huntington's disease (HD) [126,127]. However, occasional cases of HD developing at a typical mid-life age present with parkinsonism as well [128,129]. Huntington disease-like 2 (HDL2) also includes parkinsonism as one of its presentation variants [130].

In the early 1900s, pathologists began reporting the unusually frequent occurrence of an amyotrophic lateral sclerosis (ALS)-like illness (lytico) in the indigenous Chamorro population on the western Pacific island of Guam. Often lumped with lytico owing to clinical, familial, and pathological associations, is the parkinsonism-dementia complex of Guam (PDCG), known locally as bodig; 40% of patients with bodig also have lytico. PDCG has its onset in middle life, at a slightly older age for men (age 60 years) than women (age 50 years) [131]. The parkinsonism of PDCG has a typically symmetrical onset, and is predominantly akinetic in nature and unresponsive to levodopa. Although either syndrome can occur alone, parkinsonism and dementia coexist in 90% of patients. Steele and colleagues have also described PSP-like and CBD-like variants among the same population [132]. Despite a familial predisposition consistent with autosomal dominant inheritance in a majority of cases and identification of microtubule-associated protein tau (MAPT) gene polymorphisms conferring increased risk [133], investigators appear to favor an environmental etiology, largely owing

Table 6.6 Degenerative diseases causing parkinsonism

Alzheimer's disease [298]
Amyotrophic lateral sclerosis with dementia [299]
Argyrophilic grain disease [300]
Basophilic inclusion body disease [301]
Frontotemporal dementia and parkinsonism
Frontotemporal lobar degeneration with microtubule-associated protein tau gene mutation [140]
Frontotemporal lobar degeneration with tau-negative ubiquitin-positive inclusions (FTLD-U) [142]
Frontotemporal lobar degeneration with progranulin gene mutation [140]
Hereditary motor and sensory neuropathy with parkinsonism [302]
Hereditary pallidoluysionigral degeneration and amyotrophic lateral sclerosis [303]
Hereditary spastic paraplegia [304]
Hereditary spastic paraplegia with thin corpus callosum [305]
Huntington's disease [126,127]
Huntington disease-like 2 [130]
Myotonic dystrophy [306]
Neuroacanthocytosis [307]
Neuronal intermediate filament inclusion disease [308]
Pallidoluysian atrophy [309]
Perry syndrome [310]
Pick's disease [142]
Regional atypical parkinsonism (see text)
Parkinsonism-dementia complex of Guam
Kii peninsula
Irian Jaya (West Papua), New Guinea
Guadeloupe
Spinocerebellar ataxias (see text)
Thalamo-olivary degeneration [311]
X-linked recessive dystonia-parkinsonism [312]
X-linked recessive parkinsonism and mental retardation [313]

to the rapid decline in incidence in recent years [134], as well as the rare development of PDCG in immigrants to Guam.

In the 1950s, a disease with many similar clinical and pathological features was found with high prevalence in two villages in the Kii peninsula of Japan, more than 2000 km from Guam. Although early clinical accounts were dominated by an ALS-like illness (Muro disease), few patients have pure motor neuron disease, and parkinsonism and dementia are each found in over 75% of cases. Levodopa-unresponsive akinesia, rigidity, and postural instability occur more often than tremor. Variant presentations such as PSP have not been described. In contrast to PDCG, the incidence of Muro disease has not declined, and investigators in Japan favor a genetic etiology [135]. A third focus for combined ALS and the parkinsonism-dementia complex in the western Pacific region was found in villages in southern Irian Jaya (also known as West Papua), on the island of New Guinea in Indonesia, in the 1960s. Among these people the disease is known as lumpu. It shares the relative homogeneity of clinical presentation of Muro disease, but epidemiologically it is more akin to PDCG and has almost disappeared [136]. A fourth region of high prevalence of atypical parkinsonism (AP) is found on the island of Guadeloupe, on the border between the Caribbean Sea and the Atlantic Ocean. Here there is a mixture of syndromes with parkinsonism including typical PD, a PSP-like presentation, and a third clinical group termed unclassifiable [137]. In the latter two patient groups a frontal-type dementia is common, but motor neuron disease is not. Although unresponsive to levodopa, the PSP-like patients differ from those with classical PSP in the finding of features more characteristic of Lewy body diseases: tremor, hallucinations, dysautonomia, and REM-sleep behavior disorder. They also frequently exhibit cortical myoclonus and cortical ocular motor deficits predominantly [138]. However, limited pathological findings have been consistent with PSP. It has been suggested that the PSP-like and unclassifiable patients differ only in the presence or absence of oculomotor dysfunction [139], and that together they represent a distinct clinical entity not found elsewhere to date. Etiological speculation has focused on dietary consumption of Annonaceae fruit containing annonacin, a complex I inhibitor.

Frontotemporal dementia and parkinsonism is a syndrome of cognitive and behavioral deterioration accompanied by parkinsonian manifestations. On the basis of genetic and pathological findings, three underlying diseases have been described. Two are familial and are known as frontotemporal lobar degeneration with microtubule-associated protein tau gene mutation and frontotemporal lobar degeneration with progranulin gene mutation [140]; the tau and progranulin genes are adjacent to each other on chromosome 17. Specific mutations correlate partially with the phenotype [141]. The third disorder is sporadic and has been called frontotemporal lobar degeneration with tau-negative ubiquitin-positive inclusions [142].

Miscellaneous causes of parkinsonism

In this final section is an assortment of disorders (Table 6.7) that did not fit other categories. Most of these represent rare disorders, or rare complications of common disorders. The main exception is psychogenic parkinsonism. Parkinsonism represents 2–8% of all psychogenic cases in movement disorder clinics [143–145]. As with other psychogenic disorders, psychogenic parkinsonism is identified clinically by finding evidence of inconsistency and incongruity. Here inconsistency means variability of clinical features when there should be none, such as the presence of a rest tremor that disappears with distraction, while incongruity refers to the property of differing from known movement disorder phenomenology, such as prolonged pauses between repetitions of alternating movements. Aside from features uncharacteristic of organic parkinsonism, patients usually exhibit other psychogenic clinical signs [146,147]. A clinical impression of psychogenic parkinsonism can be bolstered by electrophysiological recordings that detect inconsistency [148], and dopamine transporter imaging to prove integrity of the nigrostriatal tract [149].

There are many challenges to a diagnosis of psychogenic parkinsonism, not least of which is the lack of definitive diagnostic tests for PD and other organic disorders with

Table 6.7 Miscellaneous causes of parkinsonism

Anaphylaxis [314]
Antiphospholipid syndrome [79]
Behçet's disease [315]
Bone marrow transplant [316]
Burn injury [317]
CADASIL [83]
Electrical injury [318]
Hemiparkinsonism-hemiatrophy [319]
Mixed cryoglobulinemia [81]
Moyamoya disease [82]
Multiple sclerosis [320]
Paraneoplastic [321, 322]
Polyarteritis nodosa [80]
Polymyalgia rheumatica [323]
Psychogenic parkinsonism (see text)
Radiation therapy [324]
Rett syndrome [325]
Sjogren's syndrome [326]
Systemic lupus erythematosis [327]
Trauma
Peripheral injury [328]
Repeated head trauma (pugilistic) [329]
Traumatic brain injury (single event) [330,331]
Waldenstrom's macroglobulinemia [332]

parkinsonism. Benaderette and colleagues have advocated a diagnostic approach combining clinical evaluation, electrophysiological tremor recordings, and [^{123}I]-FP-CIT SPECT scanning [150]. Most authorities seem to agree that the eye of an experienced observer of parkinsonism may be the most valuable diagnostic tool of all to recognize the incongruities and inconsistencies that lead to the correct diagnosis and management of the disorder. Unfortunately, there is no definitive treatment for psychogenic parkinsonism. It requires the cumulative clinical powers of physicians to engage these patients with empathy and persuade them to accept this diagnosis. While this does not often result in complete resolution, identification of these atypical patients is important to prevent needless consultations and investigations as well as exposure to potentially deleterious and expensive treatments.

Conclusion

The majority of people who present to movement disorder clinics with parkinsonism will turn out to have PD. Many other patients will have one of the forms of AP discussed in other chapters. However, it is important for the clinician to consider alternative diagnoses, particularly treatable, potentially reversible syndromes such as drug-induced parkinsonism, hydrocephalus and other structural abnormalities, Wilson's disease, and some forms of toxic, metabolic, and infectious parkinsonism. Evaluation for alternative causes of parkinsonism includes taking a careful drug, medical, family, and occupational history, as well as imaging of the brain.

With the development of ever more powerful tools, particularly in the field of genetics, it is anticipated that our capabilities for accurate diagnosis will continue to grow. Correct identification of parkinsonian movement disorders remains the foundation on which reliable clinical research data must be built. Operating from that premise enables investigators to explain the numerous variations on the syndrome of parkinsonism outlined in this book, and to shed light on the pathogenesis of clinical manifestations of neurological disease. Ultimately, our goal is to realize the prospect of exploiting this knowledge to therapeutic advantage.

References

1. Thanvi B, Treadwell S. Drug induced parkinsonism: a common cause of parkinsonism in older people. *Postgrad Med J* 2009; **85**(1004): 322–6.
2. Modestin J, Wehrli MV, Stephan PL, et al. Evolution of neuroleptic-induced extrapyramidal syndromes under long-term neuroleptic treatment. *Schizophr Res* 2008; **100**(1–3): 97–107.
3. Alkelai A, Greenbaus L, Rigbi A, et al. Genome-wide association study of antipsychotic-induced parkinsonism severity among schizophrenia patients. *Psychopharmacology (Berl)* 2009; **206**(3): 491–9.
4. Susatia F, Fernandez HH. Drug-induced parkinsonism. *Curr Treat Options Neurol* 2009; **11**(3): 162–9.
5. Dean CE, Kuskowski MA, Caligiuri MP. Predictors of neuroleptic-induced dyskinesia and parkinsonism: the influence of measurement methods and definitions. *J Clin Psychopharmacol* 2006; **26**(6): 560–5.
6. Tinazzi M, Antonini A, Bovi T, et al. Clinical and [123I]FP-CIT SPET imaging follow-up in patients with drug-induced parkinsonism. *J Neurol* 2009; **256**(6): 910–5.
7. Llau ME, Nguyen L, Senard JM, et al. [Drug-induced parkinsonian syndromes: a 10-year experience at a regional center of pharmaco-vigilance]. *Rev Neurol (Paris)* 1994; **150**(11): 757–62.
8. Diaz-Corrales FJ, Sanz-Viedma S, Garcia-Solis D, et al. Clinical features and 123I-FP-CIT SPECT imaging in drug-induced parkinsonism and Parkinson's disease. *Eur J Nucl Med Mol Imaging* 2010; **37**(3): 556–64.
9. Kagi G, Bhatia KP, Tolosa E. The role of DAT-SPECT in movement disorders. *J Neurol Neurosurg Psychiatry* 2010; **81**(1): 5–12.
10. Lee PH, Yeo SH, Yong SW, et al. Odour identification test and its relation to cardiac 123I-metaiodobenzylguanidine in patients with drug induced parkinsonism. *J Neurol Neurosurg Psychiatry* 2007; **78**(11): 1250–2.
11. Rochon PA, Stukel TA, Sykora K, et al. Atypical antipsychotics and parkinsonism. *Arch Intern Med* 2005; **165**(16): 1882–8.
12. Cortese L, Caligiuri MP, Williams R, et al. Reduction in neuroleptic-induced movement disorders after a switch to quetiapine in patients with schizophrenia. *J Clin Psychopharmacol* 2008; **28**(1): 69–73.
13. Miller DD, Caroff SN, Davis SM, et al. Extrapyramidal side-effects of antipsychotics in a randomised trial. *Br J Psychiatry* 2008; **193**(4): 279–88.
14. Weiden PJ. EPS profiles: the atypical antipsychotics are not all the same. *J Psychiatr Pract* 2007; **13**(1): 13–24.
15. Bharadwaj R, Grover S. Parkinsonism and akathisia with quetiapine: three case reports. *J Clin Psychiatry* 2008; **69**(7): 1189–91.
16. Shin HW, Kim MJ, Kim JS, et al. Levosulpiride-induced movement disorders. *Mov Disord* 2009; **24**(15): 2249–53.

17. Briani C, Cagnin A, Chierichetti F, et al. Thiethylperazine-induced parkinsonism: in vivo demonstration of dopamine D2 receptors blockade. *Eur J Neurol* 2004; **11**(10): 709–10.

18. De Leo V, Morgante G, Musacchio MC, et al. The safety of veralipride. *Expert Opin Drug Saf* 2006; **5**(5): 695–701.

19. Esper CD, Factor SA. Failure of recognition of drug-induced parkinsonism in the elderly. *Mov Disord* 2008; **23**(3): 401–4.

20. Van Gerpen JA. Drug-induced parkinsonism. *Neurologist* 2002; **8**(6): 363–70.

21. Teive HA, Troiano AR, Germiniani FM, et al. Flunarizine and cinnarizine-induced parkinsonism: a historical and clinical analysis. *Parkinsonism Relat Disord* 2004; **10**(4): 243–5.

22. Langston JW, Ballard P, Tetrud JW, et al. Chronic Parkinsonism in humans due to a product of meperidine-analog synthesis. *Science* 1983; **219**(4587): 979–80.

23. Watanabe Y, Himeda T, Araki T. Mechanisms of MPTP toxicity and their implications for therapy of Parkinson's disease. *Med Sci Monit* 2005; **11**(1): RA17–23.

24. Broussolle E, Thobois S. [Genetics and environmental factors of Parkinson disease]. *Rev Neurol (Paris)* 2002; **158**(Spec 1): S11–23.

25. Chade AR, Kasten M, Tanner CM. Nongenetic causes of Parkinson's disease. *J Neural Transm Suppl* 2006; **70**: 147–51.

26. Bjarkam CR, Nielsen MS, Glud AN, et al. Neuromodulation in a minipig MPTP model of Parkinson disease. *Br J Neurosurg* 2008; **22**(Suppl 1): S9–12.

27. Couper J. On the effects of black oxide of manganese when inhaled into the lungs. *Br Ann Med Pharmacol* 1837; **1**: 41–2.

28. Olanow CW. Manganese-induced parkinsonism and Parkinson's disease. *Ann NY Acad Sci* 2004; **1012**: 209–23.

29. Yamada M, Ohno S, Okayasu I, et al. Chronic manganese poisoning: a neuropathological study with determination of manganese distribution in the brain. *Acta Neuropathol (Berl)* 1986; **70**(3–4): 273–8.

30. Stepens A, Logina I, Liguts V, et al. A Parkinsonian syndrome in methcathinone users and the role of manganese. *N Engl J Med* 2008; **358**(10): 1009–17.

31. Sikk K, Taba P, Haldre S, et al. Irreversible motor impairment in young addicts – ephedrone, manganism or both? *Acta Neurol Scand* 2007; **115**(6): 385–9.

32. Sikk K, Taba P, Haldre S, et al. Clinical, neuroimaging and neurophysiological features in addicts with manganese-ephedrone exposure. *Acta Neurol Scand* 2010; 121(4): 237–43.

33. Munhoz RP, Teive HA, Troiano AR, et al. Parkinson's disease and thyroid dysfunction. *Parkinsonism Relat Disord* 2004; **10**(6): 381–3.

34. Garcia-Moreno JM, Chacon-Pena J. Hypothyroidism and Parkinson's disease and the issue of diagnostic confusion. *Mov Disord* 2003; **18**(9): 1058–9.

35. Arvanitakis Z, Wilson RS, Bienias JL, et al. Diabetes and parkinsonian signs in older persons. *Alzheimer Dis Assoc Disord* 2007; **21**(2): 144–9.

36. Sedel F, Saudubray JM, Roze E, et al. Movement disorders and inborn errors of metabolism in adults: a diagnostic approach. *J Inherit Metab Dis* 2008; **31**(3): 308–18.

37. Wilson SAK. Progressive lenticular degeneration: a familial nervous disease associated with cirrhosis of the liver. *Brain* 1912; **34**: 295–509.

38. Czlonkowska A, Rodo M, Gromadzka G. Late onset Wilson's disease: therapeutic implications. *Mov Disord* 2008; **23**(6): 896–8.

39. Taly AB, Meenakshi-Sundaram S, Sinha S, et al. Wilson disease: description of 282 patients evaluated over 3 decades. *Medicine (Baltimore)* 2007; **86**(2): 112–21.

40. da Costa Mdo D, Spitz M, Bacheschi LA, et al. Wilson's disease: two treatment modalities. Correlations to pretreatment and posttreatment brain MRI. *Neuroradiology* 2009; **51**(10): 627–33.

41. Pfeiffer RF. Wilson's Disease. *Semin Neurol* 2007; **27**(2): 123–32.

42. Brewer GJ, Askari F, Lorincz MT, et al. Treatment of Wilson disease with ammonium tetrathiomolybdate: IV. Comparison of tetrathiomolybdate and trientine in a double-blind study of treatment of the neurologic presentation

of Wilson disease. *Arch Neurol* 2006; **63**(4): 521–7.

43. Jog MS, Lang AE. Chronic acquired hepatocerebral degeneration: case reports and new insights. *Mov Disord* 1995; **10**(6): 714–22.

44. Noone ML, Kumar VG, Ummer K, et al. Cirrhosis presenting as Parkinsonism. *Ann Indian Acad Neurol* 2008; **11**(3): 179–81.

45. Burkhard PR, Delavelle J, Du Pasquier R, et al. Chronic parkinsonism associated with cirrhosis: a distinct subset of acquired hepatocerebral degeneration. *Arch Neurol* 2003; **60**(4): 521–8.

46. Federico P, Zochodne DW. Reversible parkinsonism and hyperammonemia associated with portal vein thrombosis. *Acta Neurol Scand* 2001; **103**(3): 198–200.

47. Pinarbasi B, Kaymakoglu S, Matur Z, et al. Are acquired hepatocerebral degeneration and hepatic myelopathy reversible? *J Clin Gastroenterol* 2009; **43**(2): 176–81.

48. Nagatomo S, Umehara F, Hanada K, et al. Manganese intoxication during total parenteral nutrition: report of two cases and review of the literature. *J Neurol Sci* 1999; **162**(1): 102–5.

49. da Silva CJ, da Rocha AJ, Jeronymo S, et al. A preliminary study revealing a new association in patients undergoing maintenance hemodialysis: manganism symptoms and T1 hyperintense changes in the basal ganglia. *AJNR Am J Neuroradiol* 2007; **28**(8): 1474–9.

50. Demarquay G, Setiey A, Morel Y, et al. Clinical report of three patients with hereditary hemochromatosis and movement disorders. *Mov Disord* 2000; **15**(6): 1204–9.

51. Trender-Gerhard I, Sweeney MG, Schwingenschuh P, et al. Autosomal-dominant GTPCH1-deficient DRD: clinical characteristics and long-term outcome of 34 patients. *J Neurol Neurosurg Psychiatry* 2009; **80**(8): 839–45.

52. Brashear A, Dobyns WB, de Carvalho Aguiar P, et al. The phenotypic spectrum of rapid-onset dystonia-parkinsonism (RDP) and mutations in the ATP1A3 gene. *Brain* 2007; **130**(3): 828–35.

53. Baloh RH, Salavaggione E, Milbrandt J, et al. Familial parkinsonism and ophthalmoplegia from a mutation in the mitochondrial DNA helicase twinkle. *Arch Neurol* 2007; **64**(7): 998–1000.

54. Luoma P, Melberg A, Rinne JO, et al. Parkinsonism, premature menopause, and mitochondrial DNA polymerase gamma mutations: clinical and molecular genetic study. *Lancet* 2004; **364**(9437): 875–82.

55. Thyagarajan D, Bressman S, Bruno C, et al. A novel mitochondrial 12SrRNA point mutation in parkinsonism, deafness, and neuropathy. *Ann Neurol* 2000; **48**(5): 730–6.

56. Simon DK, Pulst SM, Sutton JP, et al. Familial multisystem degeneration with parkinsonism associated with the 11778 mitochondrial DNA mutation. *Neurology* 1999; **53**(8): 1787–93.

57. Horvath R, Kley RA, Lochmüller H, et al. Parkinson syndrome, neuropathy, and myopathy caused by the mutation A8344G (MERRF) in tRNALys. *Neurology* 2007; **68**(1): 56–8.

58. Dale RC, Church AJ, Surtees RA, et al. Encephalitis lethargica syndrome: 20 new cases and evidence of basal ganglia autoimmunity. *Brain* 2004; **127**(1): 21–33.

59. Dale RC, Irani SR, Brilot F, et al. N-methyl-D-aspartate receptor antibodies in pediatric dyskinetic encephalitis lethargica. *Ann Neurol* 2009; **66**(5): 704–9.

60. Lopez-Alberola R, Georgiou M, Sfakianakis GN, et al. Contemporary Encephalitis Lethargica: phenotype, laboratory findings and treatment outcomes. *J Neurol* 2009; **256**(3): 396–404.

61. Mattos JP, Rosso AL, Correa RB, et al. Movement disorders in 28 HIV-infected patients. *Arq Neuropsiquiatr* 2002; **60**(3-A): 525–30.

62. Murakami T, Nakajima M, Nakamura T, et al. Parkinsonian symptoms as an initial manifestation in a Japanese patient with acquired immunodeficiency syndrome and Toxoplasma infection. *Intern Med* 2000; **39**(12): 1111–14.

63. Bouffard JP, Mena H, Ripple M, et al. Mesencephalic cryptococcal abscesses presenting with parkinsonism as an initial manifestation of AIDS. *Mov Disord* 2003; **18**(11): 1354–7.

64. Clay PG, Adams MM. Pseudo-Parkinson disease secondary to ritonavir-buspirone interaction. *Ann Pharmacother* 2003; **37**(2): 202–5.

65. Cardoso F. HIV-related movement disorders: epidemiology, pathogenesis and management. *CNS Drugs* 2002; **16**(10): 663–8.

66. de Rosso AL, de Mattos JP, Correa RB, et al. Parkinsonism and AIDS: a clinical comparative study before and after HAART. *Arq Neuropsiquiatr* 2009; **67**(3B): 827–30.

67. Kobylecki C, Sylverdale MA, Varma A, et al. HIV-associated Parkinsonism with levodopa-induced dyskinesia and response to highly-active antiretroviral therapy. *Mov Disord* 2009; **24**(16): 2441–2.

68. Tisch S, Brew B. Parkinsonism in HIV-infected patients on highly active antiretroviral therapy. *Neurology* 2009; **73**(5): 401–3.

69. Sejvar JJ, Haddad MB, Tierney BC, et al. Neurologic manifestations and outcome of West Nile virus infection. *JAMA* 2003; **290**(4): 511–15.

70. Beleza P, Soares-Fernandes J, Jordão MJ, et al. From juvenile parkinsonism to encephalitis lethargica, a new phenotype of post-streptococcal disorders: case report. *Eur J Paediatr Neurol* 2008; **12**(6): 505–7.

71. Sa DS, Teive HA, Troiano AR, et al. Parkinsonism associated with neurocysticercosis. *Parkinsonism Relat Disord* 2005; **11**(1): 69–72.

72. López IC, Bermejo PG, Espiga PJ, et al. [L-dopa sensitive Parkinsonism in neurocysticercosis]. *Neurologia* 2008; **23**(2): 119–21.

73. Prashantha DK, Netravathi M, Ravishankar S, et al. Reversible parkinsonism following ventriculoperitoneal shunt in a patient with obstructive hydrocephalus secondary to intraventricular neurocysticercosis. *Clin Neurol Neurosurg* 2008; **110**(7): 718–21.

74. Averbuch-Heller L, Paulson GW, Daroff RB, et al. Whipple's disease mimicking progressive supranuclear palsy: the diagnostic value of eye movement recording. *J Neurol Neurosurg Psychiatry* 1999; **66**(4): 532–5.

75. Huber FM, Bour F, Sazdovitch V, et al. Creutzfeldt–Jakob disease with slow progression. A mimicry of progressive supranuclear palsy. *Bull Soc Sci Med Grand Duche Luxemb* 2007; (2): 125–30.

76. Foltynie T, Barker R, Brayne C. Vascular parkinsonism: a review of the precision and frequency of the diagnosis. *Neuroepidemiology* 2002; **21**(1): 1–7.

77. Critchley M. Arteriosclerotic parkinsonism. *Brain* 1929; **52**: 23–83.

78. Thanvi B, Lo N, Robinson T. Vascular parkinsonism – an important cause of parkinsonism in older people. Age Ageing 2005; **34**(2): 114–9.

79. Huang YC, Lyu RK, Chen ST, et al. Parkinsonism in a patient with antiphospholipid syndrome – case report and literature review. *J Neurol Sci* 2008; **267**(1–2): 166–9.

80. Kohlhaas K, Brechmann T, Vorgerd M. [Hepatitis B associated polyarteriitis nodosa with cerebral vasculitis]. *Dtsch Med Wochenschr* 2007; **132**(34–35): 1748–52.

81. Miric D, Nahum S, Jibidar H, et al. Vascular parkinsonism in an elderly woman with mixed cryoglobulinemia associated with hepatitis C infection. *J Am Geriatr Soc* 2006; **54**(11): 1798.

82. Tan EK, Chan LL, Yu GX, et al. Vascular parkinsonism in moyamoya: microvascular biopsy and imaging correlates. *Ann Neurol* 2003; **54**(6): 836–40.

83. Wegner F, Strecker K, Schwarz J, et al. Vascular parkinsonism in a CADASIL case with an intact nigrostriatal dopaminergic system. *J Neurol* 2007; **254**(12): 1743–5.

84. Dubinsky RM, Jankovic J. Progressive supranuclear palsy and a multi-infarct state. *Neurology* 1987; **37**(4): 570–6.

85. FitzGerald PM, Jankovic J. Lower body parkinsonism: evidence for vascular etiology. *Mov Disord* 1989; **4**(3): 249–60.

86. Okuda B, Kawabata K, Tachibana H, et al. Primitive reflexes distinguish vascular parkinsonism from Parkinson's disease. *Clin Neurol Neurosurg* 2008; **110**(6): 562–5.

87. Peralta C, Werner P, Holl B, et al. Parkinsonism following striatal infarcts: incidence in a prospective stroke unit cohort. *J Neural Transm* 2004; **111**(10–11): 1473–83.

88. Kalra S, Grosset DG, Benamer HT. Differentiating vascular parkinsonism from idiopathic Parkinson's disease: a systematic review. *Mov Disord* 2010; **25**(2): 149–56.

89. Zijlmans JC, Katzenschlager R, Daniel SE, et al. The L-dopa response in vascular parkinsonism. *J Neurol Neurosurg Psychiatry* 2004; **75**(4): 545–7.

90. Kovacs T, Szirmai I, Papp M. [Clinico-pathology and differential diagnosis of Binswanger's disease]. *Ideggyogy Sz* 2005; **58**(3–4): 78–87.

91. Pedroso JL, Godeiro-Junior C, Felicio AC, et al. Multi-lacunar strokes mimicking atypical parkinsonism with an unusual neuroimaging presentation: état criblé. *Arq Neuropsiquiatr* 2008; **66**(4): 906–7.

92. Sibon I, Fenelon G, Quinn NP, et al. Vascular parkinsonism. *J Neurol* 2004; **251**(5): 513–24.

93. Zijlmans JC, Daniel SE, Hughes AJ, et al. Clinicopathological investigation of vascular parkinsonism, including clinical criteria for diagnosis. *Mov Disord* 2004; **19**(6): 630–40.

94. Ohta K, Obara K. Hemiparkinsonism with a discrete lacunar infarction in the contralateral substantia nigra. *Mov Disord* 2006; **21**(1): 124–5.

95. Akyol A, Akyildiz UO, Tataroglu C. Vascular Parkinsonism: a case of lacunar infarction localized to mesencephalic substantia nigra. *Parkinsonism Relat Disord* 2006; **12**(7): 459–61.

96. Orta Daniel SJ, Ulises RO. Stroke of the substance nigra and parkinsonism as first manifestation of systemic lupus erythematosus. *Parkinsonism Relat Disord* 2008; **14**(4): 367–9.

97. Padilla Parrado F, Campos Arillo VM, Martinez del Valle Torres MD, et al. [Hemiparkinsonism secondary to mesencephalic bleeding]. *Neurologia* 2007; **22**(7): 480–3.

98. Jenkins M, Hussain N, Lee D, et al. Reversible parkinsonism and MRI diffusion abnormalities in cortical venous thrombosis. *Neurology* 2001; **57**(2): 364–6.

99. Alp R, Alp SI, Ure H. Cavernous hemangioma: a rare cause for secondary parkinsonism: a case report. *Int J Neurosci* 2009; **119**(11): 2112–17.

100. Vhora S, Kobayashi S, Okudera H. Pineal cavernous angioma presenting with Parkinsonism. *J Clin Neurosci* 2001; **8**(3): 263–6.

101. Nogueira RG, Baccin CE, Rabinov JD, et al. Reversible parkinsonism after treatment of dural arteriovenous fistula. *J Neuroimaging* 2009; **19**(2): 183–4.

102. Kim MJ, Chung SJ, Sung YH, et al. Levodopa-responsive parkinsonism associated with hydrocephalus. *Mov Disord* 2006; **21**(8): 1279–81.

103. Kinugawa K, Itti E, Lepeintre JF, et al. Subacute dopa-responsive Parkinsonism after successful surgical treatment of aqueductal stenosis. *Mov Disord* 2009; **24**(16): 2438–40.

104. Stolze H, Kuhtz-Buschbeck JP, Drucke H, et al. Comparative analysis of the gait disorder of normal pressure hydrocephalus and Parkinson's disease. *J Neurol Neurosurg Psychiatry* 2001; **70**(3): 289–97.

105. Morishita T, Foote KD, Okun MS. INPH and Parkinson disease: differentiation by levodopa response. *Nat Rev Neurol* **6**(1): 52–6.

106. Akiguchi I, Ishii M, Watanabe Y, et al. Shunt-responsive parkinsonism and reversible white matter lesions in patients with idiopathic NPH. *J Neurol* 2008; **255**(9): 1392–9.

107. Eide PK, Sorteberg W. Diagnostic intracranial pressure monitoring and surgical management in idiopathic normal pressure hydrocephalus: a 6-year review of 214 patients. *Neurosurgery* 2010; **66**(1): 80–91.

108. Kiefer M, Meier U, Eymann R. Does idiopathic normal pressure hydrocephalus always mean a poor prognosis? *Acta Neurochir Suppl* 2010; **106**: 101–6.

109. Ishikawa, M. [Idiopathic normal pressure hydrocephalus – regarding the guideline in progress]. *Nippon Rinsho* 2004; **62** (Suppl): 290–4.

110. Manyam BV, Walters AS, Narla KR. Bilateral striopallidodentate calcinosis: clinical characteristics of patients seen in a registry. *Mov Disord* 2001; **16**(2): 258–64.

111. Manyam, B.V. What is and what is not "Fahr's disease." *Parkinsonism Relat Disord* 2005; **11**(2): 73–80.

112. Kim TW, Park IS, Kim SH, et al. Striopallidodentate calcification and progressive supranuclear palsy-like phenotype in a patient with idiopathic

hypoparathyroidism. *J Clin Neurol* 2007; **3**(1): 57–61.

113. Abe S, Tojo K, Ichida K, et al. A rare case of idiopathic hypoparathyroidism with varied neurological manifestations. *Intern Med* 1996; **35**(2): 129–34.

114. Abrey LE, Waters CH. Basal ganglia calcification after mumps encephalitis. *Mov Disord* 1996; **11**(6): 755–6.

115. Wakabayashi K, Takahashi H. [Pathology of familial Parkinson's disease]. *Brain Nerve* 2007; **59**(8): 851–64.

116. Furtado S, Payami H, Lockhart PJ, et al. Profile of families with parkinsonism-predominant spinocerebellar ataxia type 2 (SCA2). *Mov Disord* 200; **19**(6): 622–9.

117. Lu CS, Wu Chou YH, Kuo PC, et al. The parkinsonian phenotype of spinocerebellar ataxia type 2. *Arch Neurol* 2004; **61**(1): 35–8.

118. Lu CS, Chang HC, Kuo PC, et al. The parkinsonian phenotype of spinocerebellar ataxia type 3 in a Taiwanese family. *Parkinsonism Relat Disord* 2004; **10**(6): 369–73.

119. Khan NL, Giunti P, Sweeney MG, et al. Parkinsonism and nigrostriatal dysfunction are associated with spinocerebellar ataxia type 6 (SCA6). *Mov Disord* 2005; **20**(9): 1115–19.

120. Wu YR, Lin HY, Chen CM, et al. Genetic testing in spinocerebellar ataxia in Taiwan: expansions of trinucleotide repeats in SCA8 and SCA17 are associated with typical Parkinson's disease. *Clin Genet* 2004; **65**(3): 209–14.

121. Cho JW, Kim SY, Park SS, et al. Spinocerebellar ataxia type 12 was not found in Korean Parkinsonian patients. *Can J Neurol Sci* 2008; **35**(4): 488–90.

122. Lin IS, Wu RM, Lee-Chen GJ, et al. The SCA17 phenotype can include features of MSA-C, PSP and cognitive impairment. *Parkinsonism Relat Disord* 2007; **13**(4): 246–9.

123. Modoni A, Contarino MF, Bentivoglio AR, et al. Prevalence of spinocerebellar ataxia type 2 mutation among Italian Parkinsonian patients. *Mov Disord* 2007; **22**(3): 324–7.

124. Tan EK, Tong J, Pavanni R, et al. Genetic analysis of SCA 2 and 3 repeat expansions in essential tremor and atypical Parkinsonism. *Mov Disord* 2007; **22**(13): 1971–4.

125. Factor SA, Qian J, Lava NS, et al. False-positive SCA8 gene test in a patient with pathologically proven multiple system atrophy. *Ann Neurol* 2005; **57**(3): 462–3.

126. Wojaczynska-Stanek K, Adamek D, Marszal E, et al. Huntington disease in a 9-year-old boy: clinical course and neuropathologic examination. *J Child Neurol* 2006; **21**(12): 1068–73.

127. Geevasinga N, Richards FH, Jones KJ, et al. Juvenile Huntington disease. *J Paediatr Child Health* 2006; **42**(9): 552–4.

128. Wang SC, Lee-Chen GJ, Wang CK, et al. Markedly asymmetrical parkinsonism as a leading feature of adult-onset Huntington's disease. *Mov Disord* 2004; **19**(7): 854–6.

129. Reuter I, Hu MT, Andrews TC, et al. Late onset levodopa responsive Huntington's disease with minimal chorea masquerading as Parkinson plus syndrome. *J Neurol Neurosurg Psychiatry* 2000; **68**(2): 238–41.

130. Bardien S, Abrahams F, Soodyall H, et al. A South African mixed ancestry family with Huntington disease-like 2: clinical and genetic features. *Mov Disord* 2007; **22**(14): 2083–9.

131. Elizan TS, Hirano A, Abrams BM, et al. Amyotrophic lateral sclerosis and parkinsonism-dementia complex of Guam. Neurological reevaluation. *Arch Neurol* 1966; **14**(4): 356–68.

132. Steele JC. Parkinsonism-dementia complex of Guam. *Mov Disord* 2005; **20**(Suppl 12): S99–107.

133. Sundar PD, Yu CE, Sieh W, et al. Two sites in the MAPT region confer genetic risk for Guam ALS/PDC and dementia. *Hum Mol Genet* 2007; **16**(3): 295–306.

134. Plato CC, Garruto RM, Galasko D, et al. Amyotrophic lateral sclerosis and parkinsonism-dementia complex of Guam: changing incidence rates during the past 60 years. *Am J Epidemiol* 2003; **157**(2): 149–57.

135. Kuzuhara S, Kokubo Y. Atypical parkinsonism of Japan: amyotrophic lateral sclerosis-parkinsonism-dementia complex of the Kii peninsula of Japan (Muro disease): an update. *Mov Disord* 2005; **20**(Suppl 12): S108–13.

136. Spencer PS, Palmer VS, Ludolph AC. On the decline and etiology of high-incidence motor system disease in West Papua (southwest New Guinea). *Mov Disord* 2005; **20**(Suppl 12): S119–26.

137. Caparros-Lefebvre D, Lees AJ. Atypical unclassifiable parkinsonism on Guadeloupe: an environmental toxic hypothesis. *Mov Disord* 2005; **20**(Suppl 12): S114–18.

138. Apartis E, Gaymard B, Verhaeghe S, et al. Predominant cortical dysfunction in Guadeloupean parkinsonism. *Brain* 2008; **131**(10): 2701–9.

139. Lannuzel A, Hoglinger GU, Verhaeghe S, et al. Atypical parkinsonism in Guadeloupe: a common risk factor for two closely related phenotypes? *Brain* 2007; **130**(3): 816–27.

140. Tsuboi, Y. [Clinical, pathological, and genetic characteristics of frontotemporal dementia and parkinsonism linked to chromosome 17 with mutations in the MAPT and PGRN]. *Brain Nerve* 2009; **61**(11): 1285–91.

141. Ludolph AC, Kassubek J, Landwehrmeyer BG, et al. Tauopathies with parkinsonism: clinical spectrum, neuropathologic basis, biological markers, and treatment options. *Eur J Neurol* 2009; **16**(3): 297–309.

142. Yokota O, Tsuchiya K, Arai T, et al. Clinicopathological characterization of Pick's disease versus frontotemporal lobar degeneration with ubiquitin/TDP-43-positive inclusions. *Acta Neuropathol* 2009; **117**(4): 429–44.

143. Yokota O, Tsuchiya K, Arai T, et al. Clinical characteristics of 49 patients with psychogenic movement disorders in a tertiary clinic in Turkey. *Mov Disord* 2009; **24**(5): 759–62.

144. Fahn S, Williams DT. Psychogenic dystonia. *Adv Neurol* 1988; **50**: 431–55.

145. Sa DS, Galvez-Jimenez N, Lang AE. Psychogenic movement disorders. In: *Movement Disorders: Neurologic Principles & Practice*. Watts RL, Koller WC, eds. New York: McGraw-Hill, 2004; 891–914.

146. Lang AE, Koller WC, Fahn S. Psychogenic parkinsonism. *Arch Neurol* 1995; **52**(8): 802–10.

147. Factor SA, Podskalny GD, Molho ES. Psychogenic movement disorders: frequency, clinical profile, and characteristics. *J Neurol Neurosurg Psychiatry* 1995; **59**(4): 406–12.

148. Zeuner KE, Shoge RO, Goldstein SR, et al. Accelerometry to distinguish psychogenic from essential or parkinsonian tremor. *Neurology* 2003; **61**(4): 548–50.

149. Tolosa E, Coelho M, Gallardo M. DAT imaging in drug-induced and psychogenic parkinsonism. *Mov Disord* 2003; **18**(Suppl 7): S28–33.

150. Benaderette S, Zanotti Fregonara P, Apartis E, et al. Psychogenic parkinsonism: a combination of clinical, electrophysiological, and [(123)I]-FP-CIT SPECT scan explorations improves diagnostic accuracy. *Mov Disord* 2006; **21**(3): 310–17.

151. Strang RR. Parkinsonism occurring during methyldopa therapy. *Can Med Assoc J* 1966; **95**(18): 928–9.

152. Dotti MT, Federico A. Amiodarone-induced parkinsonism: a case report and pathogenetic discussion. *Mov Disor* 1995; **10**(2): 233–4.

153. Thornton JE, Stahl SM. Case report of tardive dyskinesia and parkinsonism associated with amoxapine therapy. *Am J Psychiatry* 1984; **141**(5): 704–5.

154. Manley TJ, Chusid MJ, Rand SD, et al. Reversible parkinsonism in a child after bone marrow transplantation and lipid-based amphotericin B therapy. *Pediatr Infect Dis J* 1998; **17**(5): 433–4.

155. Marti Masso JF, Carrera N, Urtasun M. Drug-induced parkinsonism: a growing list. *Mov Disord* 1993; **8**(1): 125.

156. Fox JH, Bennett DA, Goetz CG, et al. Induction of parkinsonism by intraventricular bethanechol in a patient with Alzheimer's disease. *Neurology* 1989; **39**(9): 1265.

157. Prodan CI, Monnot M, Ross ED, et al. Reversible dementia with parkinsonian features associated with budesonide use. *Neurology* 2006; **67**(4): 723.

158. Grandas F, Lopez-Manzanares L. Bupropion-induced parkinsonism. *Mov Disord* 2007; **22**(12): 1830–1.

159. Garcia-Ruiz PJ, Javier Jimenez-Jimenez F, Garcia de Yebenes J. Calcium channel

blocker-induced parkinsonism: clinical features and comparisons with Parkinson's disease. *Parkinsonism Relat Disord* 1998; **4**(4): 211–214.

160. Teive HA, Germiniani FM, Werneck LC. Parkinsonian syndrome induced by amlodipine: case report. *Mov Disord* 2002; **17**(4): 833–5.

161. Fabiani G, Pastro PC, Froehner C. Parkinsonism and other movement disorders in outpatients in chronic use of cinnarizine and flunarizine. *Arq Neuropsiquiatr* 2004; **62**(3B): 784–8.

162. Remblier C, Kassir A, Richard D, et al. [Parkinson syndrome from diltiazem]. *Therapie* 2001; **56**(1): 57–9.

163. Padrell MD, Navarro M, Faura CC, et al. Verapamil-induced parkinsonism. *Am J Med* 1995; **99**(4): 436.

164. Sandyk R. Parkinsonism induced by captopril. *Clin Neuropharmacol* 1985; **8**(2): 197–8.

165. Ross RT. Drug-induced parkinsonism and other movement disorders. *Can J Neurol Sci* 1990; **17**(2): 155–62.

166. Kenney C, Hunter C, Jankovic J. Long-term tolerability of tetrabenazine in the treatment of hyperkinetic movement disorders. *Mov Disord* 2007; **22**(2): 193–7.

167. Mintz U, Liberman UA, de Vries A. Parkinsonism syndrome due to cephaloridine. *JAMA* 1971; **216**(7): 1200.

168. Parmar RC, Valvi CV, Kamat JR, et al. Chloroquine induced parkinsonism. *J Postgrad Med* 2000; **46**(1): 29–30.

169. Handler CE, Besse CP, Wilson AO. Extrapyramidal and cerebellar syndrome with encephalopathy associated with cimetidine. *Postgrad Med J* 1982; **58**(682): 527–8.

170. Lima MA, Maradei S, Maranhao Filho P. Cyclosporine-induced parkinsonism. *J Neurol* 2009; **256**(4): 674–5.

171. Chutorian AM, Bojko A, Heier L, et al. Toxic pediatric parkinsonism: report of a child with metabolic studies and response to treatment. *J Child Neurol* 2003; **18**(11): 812–15.

172. Sandyk R. Parkinsonism induced by diazepam. *Biol Psychiatry* 1986; **21**(12): 1232–3.

173. Sato S, Nakamura K, Nakahara T, et al. [Distigmine bromide induced

Parkinsonism. A case report]. *Rinsho Shinkeigaku* 2005; **45**(8): 600–2.

174. de Mari M, De Blasi R, Lamberti P, et al. Unilateral pallidal lesion after acute disulfiram intoxication: a clinical and magnetic resonance study. *Mov Disord* 1993; **8**(2): 247–9.

175. Laplane D, Attal N, Sauron B, et al. Lesions of basal ganglia due to disulfiram neurotoxicity. *J Neurol Neurosurg Psychiatry* 1992; **55**(10): 925–9.

176. Bergevin PR, Patwardhan VC, Weissman J, et al. Letter: Neurotoxicity of 5-fluorouracil. *Lancet* 1975; **1**(7903): 410.

177. Wilson WL, Bisel HF, Cole D, et al. Prolonged low-dosage administration of hexamethylmelamine (NC 13875). *Cancer* 1970; **25**(3): 568–70.

178. Raison CL, Demetrashvili M, Capuron L, et al. Neuropsychiatric adverse effects of interferon-alpha: recognition and management. *CNS Drugs* 2005; **19**(2): 105–23.

179. Zesiewicz TA, Sanchez-Ramos J, Sullivan KL, et al. Levetiracetam-induced parkinsonism in a Huntington disease patient. *Clin Neuropharmacol* 2005; **28**(4): 188–90.

180. Walrave TR, Bulens C. [Parkinsonism during lithium use]. *Tijdschr Psychiatr* 2009; **51**(2): 123–7.

181. Dallocchio C, Mazzarello P. A case of Parkinsonism due to lithium intoxication: treatment with Pramipexole. *J Clin Neurosci* 2002; **9**(3): 310–1.

182. Olive JM, Masana L, Gonzalez J. Meperidine and reversible parkinsonism. *Mov Disord* 1994; **9**(1): 115–6.

183. Papapetropoulos S, Argyriou AA, Liossis SN, et al. A case of L-dopa-responsive parkinsonian syndrome after low-dose oral methotrexate intake. *Clin Neuropharmacol* 2004; **27**(2): 95–8.

184. Muraoka T, Oku E, Sugataka K, et al. A case of severe parkinsonism associated with short-term treatment with milnacipran. *Clin Neuropharmacol* 2008; **31**(5): 299–300.

185. Bhanji NH, Margolese HC. Extrapyramidal symptoms related to adjunctive nizatidine therapy in an adolescent receiving quetiapine and paroxetine. *Pharmacotherapy* 2004; **24**(7): 923–5.

186. Espay AJ. Reversible parkinsonism and ataxia associated with high-dose octreotide. *Neurology* 2008; **70**(24): 2345–6.

187. Serrano-Duenas M. [Parkinsonism or Parkinson's disease unmasked by pentoxifylline?] *Neurologia* 2001; **16**(1): 39–42.

188. Gordon M, Gordon AS. Perhexiline maleate as a cause of reversible parkinsonism and peripheral neuropathy. *J Am Geriatr Soc* 1981; **29**(6): 259–62.

189. Gillman MA, Sandyk R. Parkinsonism induced by a monoamine oxidase inhibitor. *Postgrad Med J* 1986; **62**(725): 235–6.

190. Ertan S, Ulu MO, Hanimoglu H, et al. Phenytoin-induced parkinsonism. *Singapore Med J* 2006; **47**(11): 981–3.

191. Perez Lloret S, Amaya M, Merello M. Pregabalin-induced parkinsonism: a case report. *Clin Neuropharmacol* 2009; **32**(6): 353–4.

192. Varenne A. [Letter: Prenylamine and parkinsonian manifestations]. *Nouv Presse Med* 1975; **4**(28): 2044.

193. Gjerris F. Transitory procaine-induced Parkinsonism. *J Neurol Neurosurg Psychiatry* 1971; **34**(1): 20–2.

194. Matsuo H, Matsui A, Nasu R, et al. Propiverine-induced Parkinsonism: a case report and a pharmacokinetic/ pharmacodynamic study in mice. *Pharm Res* 2000; **17**(5): 565–71.

195. Iwasaki Y, Kinoshita M, Wakata N. [A case report of pyridostigmine induced parkinsonism]. *Rinsho Shinkeigaku* 1988; **28**(6): 662–4.

196. Christodoulou C, Papadopoulou A, Rizos E, et al. Extrapyramidal side effects and suicidal ideation under fluoxetine treatment: a case report. *Ann Gen Psychiatry* 2010; **9**: 5.

197. Kuloglu M, Caykoylu A, Ekinci O, et al. Successful management of depression with reboxetine in a patient who developed parkinsonism related to paroxetine use. *J Psychopharmacol* 2010; 24(4): 623–4.

198. Mendhekar DN, Benuiwal RP, Puri V. Parkinsonism and elevated lactic acid with sertraline. *Can J Psychiatry* 2005; **50**(5): 301.

199. Fukunishi I, Kitaoka T, Shirai T, et al. A hemodialysis patient with trazodone-induced parkinsonism. *Nephron* 2002; **90**(2): 222–3.

200. Masmoudi K, Gras-Champel V, Douadi Y, et al. [Trimetazidine-a new aetiology for extrapyramidal disorders: A case of parkinsonism and akathisia]. *Therapie* 2005; **60**(6): 603–5.

201. Marti Masso JF, Marti I, Carrera N, et al. Trimetazidine induces parkinsonism, gait disorders and tremor. *Therapie* 2005; **60**(4): 419–22.

202. Jamora D, Lim SH, Pan A, et al. Valproate-induced Parkinsonism in epilepsy patients. *Mov Disord* 2007; **22**(1): 130–3.

203. Deahl M. Betel nut-induced extrapyramidal syndrome: an unusual drug interaction. *Mov Disord* 1989; **4**(4): 330–2.

204. Choi IS. Parkinsonism after carbon monoxide poisoning. *Eur Neurol* 2002; **48**(1): 30–3.

205. May EF, Ling GS, Geyer CA, et al. Contrast agent overdose causing brain retention of contrast, seizures and parkinsonism. *Neurology* 1993; **43**(4): 836–8.

206. Di Filippo M, Tambasco N, Muzi G, et al. Parkinsonism and cognitive impairment following chronic exposure to potassium cyanide. *Mov Disord* 2008; **23**(3): 468–70.

207. Kuoppamaki M, Rothwell JC, Brown RG, et al. Parkinsonism following bilateral lesions of the globus pallidus: performance on a variety of motor tasks shows similarities with Parkinson's disease. *J Neurol Neurosurg Psychiatry* 2005; **76**(4): 482–90.

208. Luijckx GJ, Nieuwhof C, Troost J, et al. Parkinsonism in alcohol withdrawal: case report and review of the literature. *Clin Neurol Neurosurg* 1995; **97**(4): 336–9.

209. Reddy NJ, Lewis LD, Gardner TB, et al. Two cases of rapid onset Parkinson's syndrome following toxic ingestion of ethylene glycol and methanol. *Clin Pharmacol Ther* 2007; **81**(1): 114–21.

210. Thrash B, Uthayathas S, Karuppagounder SS, et al. Paraquat and maneb induced neurotoxicity. *Proc West Pharmacol Soc* 2007; **50**: 31–42.

211. Sechi GP, Agnetti V, Piredda M, et al. Acute and persistent parkinsonism after use of diquat. *Neurology* 1992; **42**(1): 261–3.

212. da Costa Mdo D, Goncalves LR, Barbosa ER, et al. [Neuroimaging abnormalities

in parkinsonism: study of five cases]. *Arq Neuropsiquiatr* 2003; **61**(2B): 381–6.

213. Matzler W, Nagele T, Gasser T, et al. Acute parkinsonism with corresponding lesions in the basal ganglia after heroin abuse. *Neurology* 2007; **68**(6): 414.

214. Inoue N. [Extrapyramidal syndrome induced by chemical substances]. *Nippon Rinsho* 1993; **51**(11): 2924–8.

215. Meseguer E, Taboada R, Sanchez V, et al. Life-threatening parkinsonism induced by kava-kava. *Mov Disord* 2002; **17**(1): 195–6.

216. Huang CC. Parkinsonism induced by chronic manganese intoxication – an experience in Taiwan. *Chang Gung Med J* 2007; **30**(5): 385–95.

217. Miller K, Ochudlo S, Opala G, et al. [Parkinsonism in chronic occupational metallic mercury intoxication]. *Neurol Neurochir Pol* 2003; **37**(Suppl 5): 31–8.

218. Christine CW, Langston JW, Turner RS, et al. The neurophysiology and effect of deep brain stimulation in a patient with 1-methyl-4-phenyl-1,2,3,6-tetrahydropyridine-induced parkinsonism. *J Neurosurg* 2009; **110**(2): 234–8.

219. Huang CC, Yen TC, Shih TS, et al. Dopamine transporter binding study in differentiating carbon disulfide induced parkinsonism from idiopathic parkinsonism. *Neurotoxicology* 2004; **25**(3): 341–7.

220. Vanacore N, Gasparini M, Brusa L, et al. A possible association between exposure to n-hexane and parkinsonism. *Neurol Sci* 2000; **21**(1): 49–52.

221. Uitti RJ, Snow BJ, Shinotoh H, et al. Parkinsonism induced by solvent abuse. *Ann Neurol* 1994; **35**(5): 616–19.

222. Gash DM, Rutland K, Hudson NL, et al. Trichloroethylene: Parkinsonism and complex 1 mitochondrial neurotoxicity. *Ann Neurol* 2008; **63**(2): 184–92.

223. Gralewicz S, Dyzma M. Organic solvents and the dopaminergic system. *Int J Occup Med Environ Health* 2005; **18**(2): 103–13.

224. Hageman G, van der Hoek J, van Hout M, et al. Parkinsonism, pyramidal signs, polyneuropathy, and cognitive decline after long-term occupational solvent exposure. *J Neurol* 1999; **246**(3): 198–206.

225. Shahar E, Bentur Y, Bar-Joseph G, et al. Extrapyramidal parkinsonism complicating acute organophosphate insecticide poisoning. *Pediatr Neurol* 2005; **33**(5): 378–82.

226. McCrank E. Parkinsonism secondary to petroleum exposure. *Neurology* 1995; **45**(11): 2112.

227. Berg D, Hochstrasser H. Iron metabolism in Parkinsonian syndromes. *Mov Disord* 2006; **21**(9): 1299–310.

228. Ferrara J, Jankovic J. Acquired hepatocerebral degeneration. *J Neurol* 2009; **256**(3): 320–32.

229. Aggarwal A, Vaidya S, Shah S, et al. Reversible Parkinsonism and T1W pallidal hyperintensities in acute liver failure. *Mov Disord* 2006; **21**(11): 1986–90.

230. Friedman JH, Ambler M. Progressive parkinsonism associated with Rosenthal fibers: senile-onset alexander's disease? *Neurology* 1992; **42**(9): 1733–5.

231. Miao J, Su C, Wang W, et al. Delayed parkinsonism with a selective symmetric basal ganglia lesion after manual strangulation. *J Clin Neurosci* 2009; **16**(4): 573–5.

232. Sadeh M, Goldhammer Y. Extrapyramidal syndrome responsive to dopaminergic treatment following recovery from central pontine myelinolysis. *Eur Neurol* 1993; **33**(1): 48–50.

233. Su CS, Chang WN, Huang SH, et al. Cerebrotendinous xanthomatosis patients with and without parkinsonism: clinical characteristics and neuroimaging findings. *Mov Disord* 2010; **25**(4): 452–8.

234. Nijssen PC, Brusse E, Leyten AC, et al. Autosomal dominant adult neuronal ceroid lipofuscinosis: parkinsonism due to both striatal and nigral dysfunction. *Mov Disord* 2002; **17**(3): 482–7.

235. Sedel F, Ribeiro MJ, Remy P, et al. Dihydropteridine reductase deficiency: levodopa's long-term effectiveness without dyskinesia. *Neurology* 2006; **67**(12): 2243–5.

236. Shin HW, Song D, Sohn YH. Normal diffusion-weighted MR imaging predicts a good prognosis in extrapontine myelinolysis-induced parkinsonism. *Mov Disord* 2009; **24**(11): 1701–3.

237. Buechner S, De Cristofaro MT, Ramat S, et al. Parkinsonism and Anderson Fabry's disease: a case report. *Mov Disord* 2006; **21**(1): 103–7.

238. Clayton PT, Smith I, Harding B, et al. Subacute combined degeneration of the cord, dementia and parkinsonism due to an inborn error of folate metabolism. *J Neurol Neurosurg Psychiatry* 1986; **49**(8): 920–7.

239. Kraoua I, Stirnemann J, Ribeiro MJ, et al. Parkinsonism in Gaucher's disease type 1: ten new cases and a review of the literature. *Mov Disord* 2009; **24**(10): 1524–30.

240. Roze E, Paschke E, Lopez N, et al. Dystonia and parkinsonism in GM1 type 3 gangliosidosis. *Mov Disord* 2005; **20**(10): 1366–9.

241. Inzelberg R, Korczyn AD. Parkinsonism in adult-onset GM2 gangliosidosis. *Mov Disord* 1994; **9**(3): 375–7.

242. Gaig C, Marti MJ, Tolosa E, et al. Parkinsonism-hyperpyrexia syndrome not related to antiparkinsonian treatment withdrawal during the 2003 summer heat wave. *J Neurol* 2005; **252**(9): 1116–19.

243. Ekinci B, Apaydin H, Vural M, et al. Two siblings with homocystinuria presenting with dystonia and parkinsonism. *Mov Disord* 2004; **19**(8): 962–4.

244. Finsterer J. Parkinson syndrome as a manifestation of mitochondriopathy. *Acta Neurol Scand* 2002; **105**(5): 384–9.

245. Ekinci B, Apaydin H, Vural M, et al. Clinical features and natural history of neuroferritinopathy caused by the FTL1 460InsA mutation. *Brain* 2007; **130**(1): 110–19.

246. Seo JH, Song SK, Lee PH. A novel PANK2 mutation in a patient with atypical pantothenate-kinase-associated neurodegeneration presenting with adult-onset parkinsonism. *J Clin Neurol* 2009; **5**(4): 192–4.

247. Evans AH, Costa DC, Gacinovic S, et al. L-Dopa-responsive Parkinson's syndrome in association with phenylketonuria: In vivo dopamine transporter and D2 receptor findings. *Mov Disord* 2004; **19**(10): 1232–6.

248. Krim E, Vital A, Macia F, et al. Atypical parkinsonism combining alpha-synuclein inclusions and polyglucosan body disease. *Mov Disord* 2005; **20**(2): 200–4.

249. Mellick G, Price L, Boyle R. Late-onset presentation of pyruvate dehydrogenase deficiency. *Mov Disord* 2004; **19**(6): 727–9.

250. Zafeiriou DI, Willemsen MA, Verbeek MM, et al. Tyrosine hydroxylase deficiency with severe clinical course. *Mol Genet Metab* 2009; **97**(1): 18–20.

251. Adler CH, Stern MB, Brooks ML. Parkinsonism secondary to bilateral striatal fungal abscesses. *Mov Disord* 1989; **4**(4): 333–7.

252. Vital A, Fernagut PO, Canron MH, et al. The nigrostriatal pathway in Creutzfeldt-Jakob disease. *J Neuropathol Exp Neurol* 2009; **68**(7): 809–15.

253. Cree BC, Bernardini GL, Hays AP, et al. A fatal case of coxsackievirus B4 meningoencephalitis. *Arch Neurol* 2003; **60**(1): 107–12.

254. Poser CM, Huntley CJ, Poland JD. Para-encephalitic parkinsonism. Report of an acute case due to coxsackie virus type B2 and re-examination of the etiologic concepts of postencephalitic parkinsonism. *Acta Neurol Scand* 1969; **45**(2): 199–215.

255. Toovey S. Influenza-associated central nervous system dysfunction: a literature review. *Travel Med Infect Dis* 2008; **6**(3): 114–24.

256. Murgod UA, Muthane UB, Ravi V, et al. Persistent movement disorders following Japanese encephalitis. *Neurology* 2001; **57**(12): 2313–15.

257. Mellon AF, Appleton RE, Gardner-Medwin D, et al. Encephalitis lethargica-like illness in a five-year-old. *Dev Med Child Neurol* 1991; **33**(2): 158–61.

258. Warembourg H, Niquet G, Pauchant M, et al. [Parkinson's syndrome. Sequela of an acute poliomyelitis in the form of lethargic encephalitis in a 20-month-old child]. *Sem Hop* 1962; **38**: 2299–307.

259. Schultz DR, Barthal JS, Garrett G. Western equine encephalitis with rapid onset of parkinsonism. *Neurology* 1977; **27**(11): 1095–6.

260. Roselli F, Russo I, Fraddosio A, et al. Reversible Parkinsonian syndrome associated with anti-neuronal antibodies in acute EBV encephalitis: a case report. *Parkinsonism Relat Disord* 2006; **12**(4): 257–60.

261. Ickenstein GW, Klotz JM, Langohr HD. [Virus encephalitis with symptomatic Parkinson syndrome, diabetes insipidus

and panhypopituitarism]. *Fortschr Neurol Psychiatr* 1999; **67**(10): 476–81.

262. Misra UK, Kalita J. Prognosis of Japanese encephalitis patients with dystonia compared to those with parkinsonian features only. *Postgrad Med J* 2002; **78**(918): 238–41.

263. Pranzatelli MR, Mott SH, Pavlakis SG, et al. Clinical spectrum of secondary parkinsonism in childhood: a reversible disorder. *Pediatr Neurol* 1994; **10**(2): 131–40.

264. Provini F, Vetrugno R, Pierangeli G, et al. Sleep and temperature rhythms in two sisters with P102L Gerstmann-Straussler-Scheinker (GSS) disease. *Sleep Med* 2009; **10**(3): 374–7.

265. Haruta S, Manome T, Oguchi K, et al. [Hemiparkinsonism, probably due to malaria (author's transl)]. *Rinsho Shinkeigaku* 1978; **18**(2): 103–7.

266. Kim JS, Choi IS, Lee MC. Reversible parkinsonism and dystonia following probable mycoplasma pneumoniae infection. *Mov Disord* 1995; **10**(4): 510–12.

267. Reijneveld JC, Taphoorn MJ, Hoogenraad TU, et al. Severe but transient parkinsonism after tetanus vaccination. *J Neurol Neurosurg Psychiatry* 1997; **63**(2): 258.

268. Plesner AM, Arlien-Soborg P, Herning M. Neurological complications to vaccination against Japanese encephalitis. *Eur J Neurol* 1998; **5**(5): 479–85.

269. Jansen C, van Swieten JC, Capellari S, et al. Inherited Creutzfeldt-Jakob disease in a Dutch patient with a novel five octapeptide repeat insertion and unusual cerebellar morphology. *J Neurol Neurosurg Psychiatry* 2009; **80**(12): 1386–9.

270. Tunnell E, Wollman R, Mallik S, et al. A novel PRNP-P105S mutation associated with atypical prion disease and a rare PrPSc conformation. *Neurology* 2008; **71**(18): 1431–8.

271. O'Riordan S, McGuigan C, Farrell M, et al. Progressive multifocal leucoencephalopathy presenting with Parkinsonism. *J Neurol* 2003; **250**(11): 1379–81.

272. Sawaishi Y, Yano T, Watanabe Y, et al. Migratory basal ganglia lesions in subacute sclerosing panencephalitis (SSPE): clinical implications of axonal spread. *J Neurol Sci* 1999; **168**(2): 137–40.

273. Cubo E. [Movement disorders in adult-onset measles encephalitis]. *Neurologia* 2003; **18**(1): 30–3.

274. Spitz M, Maia FM, Gomes HR, et al. Parkinsonism secondary to neurosyphilis. *Mov Disord* 2008; **23**(13): 1948–9.

275. Kornilova Z, Khokhlov Iu K, Savin AA, et al. [Clinical aspects, diagnosis and treatment of neurological complications of tuberculosis]. *Probl Tuberk* 2001; 3: 29–32.

276. de la Fuente-Aguado J, Bordon J, Moreno JA, et al. Parkinsonism in an HIV-infected patient with hypodense cerebral lesion. *Tuber Lung Dis* 1996; **77**(2): 191–2.

277. Averbuch-Heller L, Paulson GW, Daroff RB, et al. Whipple's disease mimicking progressive supranuclear palsy: the diagnostic value of eye movement recording. *J Neurol Neurosurg Psychiatry* 1999; **66**(4): 532–5.

278. Uldry PA, Bogousslavsky J. Partially reversible parkinsonism in Whipple's disease with antibiotherapy. *Eur Neurol* 1992; **32**(3): 151–3.

279. Uldry PA, Bogousslavsky J, Petridis A, et al. Aneurysm presenting as parkinsonism. *Neurology* 2006; **67**(11): 2028.

280. Ho BL, Lieu AS, Hsu CY. Hemiparkinsonism secondary to an infiltrative astrocytoma. *Neurologist* 2008; **14**(4): 258–61.

281. Sanchez-Guerra M, Cerezal L, Leno C, et al. Primary brain lymphoma presenting as Parkinson's disease. *Neuroradiology* 2001; **43**(1): 36–40.

282. Asada T, Takayama Y, Tokuriki Y, et al. Gliomatosis cerebri presenting as a parkinsonian syndrome. *J Neuroimaging* 2007; **17**(3): 269–71.

283. Duron E, Lazareth A, Gaubert JY, et al. Gliomatosis cerebri presenting as rapidly progressive dementia and parkinsonism in an elderly woman: a case report. *J Med Case Reports* 2008; **2**: 53.

284. Bosch J, Vilalta J, Tintore M, et al. [Parkinsonian hemi-syndrome as the initial manifestation of supratentorial cystic hemangioblastoma in a patient with Von Hippel-Lindau disease]. *Rev Neurol* 1998; **26**(150): 221–3.

285. Benincasa D, Romano A, Mastronardi L, et al. Hemiparkinsonism due to frontal

meningioma. *Acta Neurol Belg* 2008; **108**(1): 29–32.

286. Bostantjopoulou S, Katsarou Z, Petridis A. Relapsing hemiparkinsonism due to recurrent meningioma. *Parkinsonism Relat Disord* 2007; **13**(6): 372–4.

287. Singer C, Schatz NJ, Bowen B, et al. Asymmetric predominantly ipsilateral blepharospasm and contralateral parkinsonism in an elderly patient with a right mesencephalic cyst. *Mov Disord* 1998; **13**(1): 135–9.

288. Pohle T, Krauss JK. Parkinsonism in children resulting from mesencephalic tumors. *Mov Disord* 1999; **14**(5): 842–6.

289. Ghaemi K, Krauss JK, Nakamura M. Hemiparkinsonism due to a pontomesencephalic cavernoma: improvement after resection. Case report. *J Neurosurg Pediatr* 2009; **4**(2): 143–6.

290. Burkhardt K, Heuberger F, Delavelle J. Pilocytic astrocytoma in the elderly. *Clin Neuropathol* 2007; **26**(6): 306–10.

291. Rondot P, Bathien N, de Recondo J, et al. Dystonia-parkinsonism syndrome resulting from a bullet injury in the midbrain. *J Neurol Neurosurg Psychiatry* 1994; **57**(5): 658.

292. Morgan JT, Scumpia AJ, Webster TM, et al. Resting tremor secondary to a pineal cyst: case report and review of the literature. *Pediatr Neurosurg* 2008; **44**(3): 234–8.

293. Dolendo MC, Lin TP, Tat OH, et al. Parkinsonism as an unusual presenting symptom of pineal gland teratoma. *Pediatr Neurol* 2003; **28**(4): 310–12.

294. Ghika J, De Tribolet N, Regli F, et al. L-dopa resistant parkinsonism in an adult woman with a cyst in the posterior fossa. *Schweiz Arch Neurol Psychiatr* 1993; **144**(5): 475–80.

295. Giray S, Sarica FB, Sen O, et al. Parkinsonian syndrome associated with subacute subdural haematoma and its effective surgical treatment: a case report. *Neurol Neurochir Pol* 2009; **43**(3): 289–92.

296. Bostantjopoulou S, Katsarou Z, Michael M, et al. Reversible parkinsonism due to chronic bilateral subdural hematomas. *J Clin Neurosci* 2009; **16**(3): 458–60.

297. Frosini D, Ceravolo R, Rossi C, et al. Bilateral thalamic glioma presenting with parkinsonism. *Mov Disord* 2009; **24**(14): 2168–9.

298. Liu Y, Stern Y, Chun MR, et al. Pathological correlates of extrapyramidal signs in Alzheimer's disease. *Ann Neurol* 1997; **41**(3): 368–74.

299. Shintaku M, Oyanagi K, Kaneda D. Amyotrophic lateral sclerosis with dementia showing clinical parkinsonism and severe degeneration of the substantia nigra: report of an autopsy case. *Neuropathology* 2007; **27**(3): 295–9.

300. Uchikado H, Tsuchiya K, Tominaga I, et al. [Argyrophilic grain disease clinically mimicking Parkinson's disease with dementia: report of an autopsy case]. *No To Shinkei* 2004; **56**(9): 785–8.

301. Yokota O, Tsuchiya K, Terada S, et al. Basophilic inclusion body disease and neuronal intermediate filament inclusion disease: a comparative clinicopathological study. *Acta Neuropathol* 2008; **115**(5): 561–75.

302. Jaradeh S, Dyck PJ. Hereditary motor and sensory neuropathy with treatable extrapyramidal features. *Arch Neurol* 1992; **49**(2): 175–8.

303. Portera-Cailliau C, Russ C, Brown RH Jr, et al. A familial form of pallidoluysionigral degeneration and amyotrophic lateral sclerosis with divergent clinical presentations. *J Neuropathol Exp Neurol* 2007; **66**(7): 650–9.

304. Goizet C, Boukhris A, Mundwiller E, et al. Complicated forms of autosomal dominant hereditary spastic paraplegia are frequent in SPG10. *Hum Mutat* 2009; **30**(2): E376–85.

305. Kang SY, Lee MH, Lee SK, et al. Levodopa-responsive parkinsonism in hereditary spastic paraplegia with thin corpus callosum. *Parkinsonism Relat Disord* 2004; **10**(7): 425–7.

306. Lim SY, Wadia P, Wenning GK, et al. Clinically probable multiple system atrophy with predominant parkinsonism associated with myotonic dystrophy type 2. *Mov Disord* 2009; **24**(9): 1407–9.

307. Bostantjopoulou S, Katsarou Z, Kazis A, et al. Neuroacanthocytosis presenting as parkinsonism. *Mov Disord* 2000; **15**(6): 1271–3.

308. Molina-Porcel L, Llado A, Rey MJ, et al. Clinical and pathological heterogeneity of neuronal intermediate filament inclusion disease. *Arch Neurol* 2008; **65**(2): 272–5.

309. Wooten GF, Lopes MB, Harris WO, et al. Pallidoluysian atrophy: dystonia and basal ganglia functional anatomy. *Neurology* 1993; **43**(9): 1764–8.

310. Wider C, Dachsel JC, Farrer MJ, et al. Elucidating the genetics and pathology of Perry syndrome. *J Neurol Sci* 2010; 289(1–2): 149–54.

311. Yamamoto T, Yamashita M. Thalamo-olivary degeneration in a patient with laryngopharyngeal dystonia. *J Neurol Neurosurg Psychiatry* 1995; **59**(4): 438–41.

312. Deng H, Le WD, Jankovic J. Genetic study of an American family with DYT3 dystonia (lubag). *Neurosci Lett* 2008; **448**(2): 180–3.

313. Gregg RG, Metzenberg AB, Hogan K, et al. Waisman syndrome, a human X-linked recessive basal ganglia disorder with mental retardation: localization to Xq27.3-qter. *Genomics* 1991; **9**(4): 701–6.

314. Garcia-Estevez DA. [Delayed anoxic-ischaemic encephalopathy: a case of Parkinsonism secondary to anaphylactic shock]. *Rev Neurol* 2009; 48(5): 271–2.

315. Joseph FG, Scolding NJ. Neuro-Behcet's disease in Caucasians: a study of 22 patients. *Eur J Neurol* 2007; **14**(2): 174–80.

316. Pavletic ZS, Bishop MR, Markopoulou K, et al. Drug-induced parkinsonism after allogeneic bone marrow transplantation. *Bone Marrow Transplant* 1996; **17**(6): 1185–7.

317. Shahar E, Keidan I, Brand N, et al. Uncommon neurologic complications of burns in infants: a parkinsonian extrapyramidal disorder and massive cerebral infarction. *J Burn Care Rehabil* 1991; **12**(1): 54–7.

318. Morris HR, Moriabadi NF, Lees AJ, et al. Parkinsonism following electrical injury to the hand. *Mov Disord* 1998; **13**(3): 600–2.

319. Silvers DS, Menkes DL. Hemibody mirror movements in hemiparkinsonism-hemiatrophy syndrome. *J Neurol Sci* 2009; **287**(1–2): 260–3.

320. Saidha S, Mok TH, Butler M, et al. Multiple sclerosis exceptionally presenting as parkinsonism responds to intravenous methylprednisolone. *J Clin Neurosci* 2010; **17**(5): 654–5.

321. Mehta SH, Morgan JC, Sethi KD. Paraneoplastic movement disorders. *Curr Neurol Neurosci Rep* 2009; **9**(4): 285–91.

322. Tan JH, Goh BC, Tambyah PA, et al. Paraneoplastic progressive supranuclear palsy syndrome in a patient with B-cell lymphoma. *Parkinsonism Relat Disord* 2005; **11**(3): 187–91.

323. Fietta P, Manganelli P. Steroid-reversible parkinsonism as presentation of polymyalgia rheumatica. *Clin Rheumatol* 2006; **25**(4): 564–5.

324. Voermans NC, Bloem BR, Janssens G, et al. Secondary parkinsonism in childhood: A rare complication after radiotherapy. *Pediatr Neurol* 2006; **34**(6): 495–8.

325. Roze E, Cochen V, Sangla S, et al. Rett syndrome: an overlooked diagnosis in women with stereotypic hand movements, psychomotor retardation, Parkinsonism, and dystonia? *Mov Disord* 2007; **22**(3): 387–9.

326. Hassin-Baer S, Levy Y, Langevitz P, et al. Anti-beta2-glycoprotein I in Sjogren's syndrome is associated with parkinsonism. *Clin Rheumatol* 2007; **26**(5): 743–7.

327. Joseph FG, Lammie GA, Scolding NJ. CNS lupus: a study of 41 patients. *Neurology* 2007; **69**(7): 644–54.

328. Jankovic J. Peripherally induced movement disorders. *Neurol Clin* 2009; **27**(3): 821–32, vii.

329. McKee AC, Cantu RC, Nowinski CJ, et al. Chronic traumatic encephalopathy in athletes: progressive tauopathy after repetitive head injury. *J Neuropathol Exp Neurol* 2009; **68**(7): 709–35.

330. Bazarian JJ, Cernak I, Noble-Haeusslein L, et al. Long-term neurologic outcomes after traumatic brain injury. *J Head Trauma Rehabil* 2009; **24**(6): 439–51.

331. Formisano R, Cicinelli P, Buzzi MG, et al. Blink reflex changes in parkinsonism following severe traumatic brain injury correlates with diffuse axonal injury. *Med Sci Monit* 2009; **15**(3): CR101–6.

332. Rudnicki SA, Harik SI, Dhodapkar M, et al. Nervous system dysfunction in Waldenstrom's macroglobulinemia: response to treatment. *Neurology* 1998; **51**(4): 1210–13.

The differential diagnosis of parkinsonism: A clinical approach

Carlo Colosimo

Introduction

The term parkinsonism is applied when a patient has a combination of tremor, bradykinesia/akinesia, rigidity, and postural instability. Parkinson's disease (PD) is by far the most common etiology of parkinsonism, accounting for up of 85% of the cases, even though other causes are not rare (Table 7.1). Although various sets of clinical diagnostic criteria are available for differentiating PD from other forms of parkinsonism, most clinical features are characterized by an inadequate sensitivity and positive predictive value in the diagnosis of these conditions [1]. PD can be recognized easily in patients with a typical presentation of cardinal signs and excellent response to dopaminergic treatment associated with drug-induced dyskinesia, whereas the differential diagnosis with other forms of parkinsonism can be challenging in other cases, particularly in the early phases of the disease. Misdiagnosis rates in clinicopathological series are relatively high, even when patients have been assessed by movement disorder specialists [2]. Indeed, several atypical cases of autopsy-documented PD resembling other disorders have been described. The use of well-defined criteria, the validity and reliability of which have been summarized in a review by the Task Force of the Movement Disorder Society [1], has improved the diagnostic accuracy of parkinsonism. However, results from a study carried out in two specialized centers in the United Kingdom and Spain showed that 4–5% of patients with parkinsonism cannot be categorized using currently available clinical diagnostic criteria for parkinsonism [3].This chapter will systematically review the motor and non-motor clinical features (Table 7.2) that may help most in the differential diagnosis of parkinsonism.

Motor symptoms
Tremor

Tremor is defined as an involuntary, rhythmic, repetitive movement of regular frequency and variable amplitude of one or more body parts. Tremor is a major issue in the diagnostic work-up for parkinsonism (Table 7.3), it being common to 80% of patients with PD; characteristically it is observed at rest, and becomes less marked or disappears with movement [4]. Rest tremor is asymmetrical, initially involving the distal upper limb before spreading to the ipsilateral lower limb after a mean of three years and to the contralateral limbs much later [5]. In addition to the classical rest tremor, many patients, particularly those with early

Handbook of Atypical Parkinsonism, eds. Carlo Colosimo, David E. Riley, and Gregor K. Wenning. Published by Cambridge University Press. © Cambridge University Press 2011.

Table 7.1 Classification of parkinsonism

Parkinson's disease
Sporadic
Familial (autosomal dominant or recessive)
Atypical parkinsonism (degenerative)
Multiple system atrophy
Progressive supranuclear palsy
Corticobasal degeneration
Dementia with Lewy bodies
Frontotemporal lobar degeneration
PARK 1 and 9 parkinsonism
Huntington's disease
Fahr's disease
Neuroacanthocytosis
Dentatorubropallidal-luysian atrophy
Prion diseases
Pantotenate-kinase associated neurodegeneration
Dopa-responsive dystonia (Segawa's disease)
Alzheimer's disease
Spinocerebellar ataxia type 2, 3 and 17
Symptomatic or secondary parkinsonism
Drug-induced
Vascular
Toxic
Metabolic (including Wilson's disease)
Obstructive and normotensive hydrocephalus
Tumors (supratentorial and brainstem)
Infectious (postencephalitic, neurosyphilis, toxoplasmosis)
Post-traumatic
Chronic subdural hematoma
Psychogenic

PD, may have concomitant or even isolated action or postural tremor. Tremor in PD has a frequency of 4–7 Hz and is enhanced by emotional stress but disappears during the deep stages of sleep [6–7]. Rest tremor is often detected more easily during gait examination: in its classic form, it is best observed in the fingers and hands of patients and is commonly

Table 7.2 Motor and non-motor symptoms of parkinsonism

Motor symptoms
Tremor
Bradykinesia
Rigidity
Postural instability
Postural deformities (camptocormia, Pisa syndrome, antecollis, retrocollis)
Gait disorders
Dysarthria and dysphagia
Oculomotor disorders (gaze-evoked nystagmus, saccadic pursuit, slow saccades, gaze palsy)
Non-motor symptoms
Olfactory dysfunction
Other sensory disturbances (including pain)
Sleep disorders (insomnia, REM-sleep behavior disorder, excessive sleepiness, inspiratory stridor)
genitourinary and skin disorders
Neuropsychiatric disorders (anxiety, depression, apathy, psychosis, dysexecutive syndrome, dementia)
Other symptoms
Fatigue
Weight loss, weight gain

Table 7.3 Tremor in parkinsonism: phenomenology

PD: unilateral or asymmetric pill-rolling rest tremor. A postural/kinetic component (re-emergent tremor) may also be present
MSA: postural/kinetic tremor frequent (~2/3 of the cases). Often incorporating myoclonus, that gives it an irregular quality ("jerky postural tremor")
PSP: uncommon, only in the PSP-P phenotype
CBD: the common myoclonic jerks of the involved limb(s) can clinically resemble tremor

described as pill-rolling. Rest tremor can also involve the jaw and tongue, often with the same frequency as in the hands, but rarely affects the head [8].

Not all rest tremors are a result of PD; indeed, rest tremors can be present in atypical parkinsonism (AP) or in essential tremor (ET) [9]. The tremor in ET is classically symmetrical and postural, although variations in the clinical pattern are common [10]. Because patients with ET sometimes display a mild increase in muscle tone, which can also be a consequence of normal aging, distinguishing PD from ET in the elderly may be challenging [10]. Useful clinical strategies to clarify the diagnosis of PD tremor include a positive clinical response to levodopa, even though tremor response to medications in PD is often unpredictable.

Unlike the tremor associated with PD, the tremor observed in two-thirds of the patients with multiple system atrophy (MSA) is of the postural or kinetic type [11]. Tremor in MSA may be accompanied by touch- and stimulus-sensitive myoclonus, which gives it an irregular quality [12,13]. Progressive supranuclear palsy (PSP), especially the classic Richardson syndrome phenotype, rarely causes tremor [14]. In the PSP parkinsonism phenotype, an asymmetrical onset of rest tremor, which responds moderately well to levodopa in the early stages, may be observed and is often confused with the tremor in PD. In corticobasal degeneration (CBD), myoclonic jerks of the limb may resemble tremor clinically. A jerky tremor is a common sign in individuals with CBD [15], whereas resting tremor is only occasionally present.

Another clinical entity that sometimes manifests itself with resting tremor is drug-induced parkinsonism (DIP), which is often indistinguishable clinically from classic PD [16]. As DIP is fairly similar to PD, a correct diagnosis requires a detailed medical history, including any information on possible exposure to agents that interfere with dopaminergic transmission. The onset of DIP differs from that of PD insofar as symptom onset may be rather abrupt in the former, often developing within weeks of drug initiation or a dose increase. Drug-induced tremor typically develops in patients treated with dopamine receptor blockers (typical and atypical antipsychotic drugs, all antiemetics except domperidone, certain calcium channel blockers such as flunarizine and cinnarizine). Besides classic resting tremor, patients with DIP may also have postural tremor. Tremor generally affects the arms more than the legs. The relative although not absolute symmetry of drug-induced tremor also helps to differentiate DIP from PD. The best way of definitively differentiating drug-induced tremors from other tremors is to suspend the presumed culprit drug and monitor the patient until the tremor disappears. Patients with pre-clinical PD, however, may be unmasked by exposure to dopamine blocking drugs.

Vascular parkinsonism (VP), a parkinsonism that occurs in patients with cerebrovascular disease, is characterized by a sudden onset and continuously progressive step-wise deterioration [17]. The resting tremor of the pill-rolling type that is characteristic of PD is typically absent, while an atypical type of resting tremor is found only in approximately 20% of possible VP cases [18]. A strategic vascular lesion in the brainstem or thalamus, unlike in VP, may determine the so-called rubral tremor [19], which is a very disabling clinical condition that responds poorly to dopaminergic therapy.

Tremor is also seen in approximately 60% of patients with Wilson's disease (WD), frequently during posture and action although rarely at rest [20]. Tremor in WD may start in one limb and then spread to the whole body. It may vary from a mild resting tremor in the fingers to marked tremor sometimes involving the entire body. The characteristic high-amplitude proximal tremor (wing-beating tremor) is best seen during arm stretching.

Bradykinesia and akinesia

Bradykinesia and/or akinesia is a central feature of all cases of parkinsonism (Table 7.4). Bradykinesia refers to slowness of voluntary movement, with a characteristic progressive reduction in speed and amplitude during repetitive actions, whereas akinesia refers to a lack

Table 7.4 Akinesia/rigidity in parkinsonism: phenomenology

PD: almost always asymmetrical
MSA: more often asymmetrical than symmetrical, but always bilateral
PSP: marked axial, minimal appendicular (in classical Richardson's syndrome)
CBD: severe and markedly asymmetrical
Vascular: in the classical "lower body" form predominantly affecting lower limbs
Wilson's disease: often asymmetrical

of spontaneous movement and delayed initiation of voluntary movement when the patient attempts to move. Bradykinesia and akinesia are different although closely related. Patients with bradykinesia have difficulty in rising from a sitting position, hesitancy in initiating walking, reduced stride length with loss of a brisk heel-strike, and a tendency to turn in several stages rather than pivoting. Like tremor, bradykinesia in PD usually begins in an upper limb, progressively spreads to the ipsilateral lower limb, and later generalizes to the contralateral side of the body [5].

Slowness of voluntary movement includes a masked facial expression with a decreased blink rate, a reduced rate of spontaneous swallowing, and a tendency not to swing the arm on the affected side(s) when walking. Bradykinesia in PD is typically responsive to dopaminergic therapy, this response being sustained over years. Unfortunately, neither the severity nor the clinical features of bradykinesia invariably helps to distinguish the different conditions with parkinsonism. Patients with AP, such as the parkinsonism variant of MSA (MSA-P), commonly have more pronounced bradykinesia than those who have had PD for the same period of time [12]. The relative symmetry of bradykinesia is a feature that distinguishes MSA-P from PD. Bradykinesia in MSA is characterized by a poor response to levodopa, even though 30–40% of patients initially exhibit a good response [13]. The symmetrical onset and rapid progression of bradykinesia are also characteristic of bradykinesia in PSP. In contrast to other conditions with parkinsonism, the bradykinesia in patients with PSP affects axial segments to a greater degree than limb segments. In occasional cases, PSP may manifest as a pure akinetic syndrome with early gait involvement associated with freezing [21]. Although few patients reap any major benefit from treatment with levodopa, approximately 30% experience some improvement at an early stage of the disease [22]. Patients with CBD may simulate PD by having marked asymmetrical bradykinesia, although these two entities can usually be distinguished by other hallmarks of CBD such as apraxia, alien limb phenomenon, slowly progressive aphasia, loss of cortical sensory function, myoclonus, and limb dystonia [23]. Dopaminergic medications do not modify features of parkinsonism in CBD [15,23].

Patients with DIP are frequently unaware of any motor problem until tremor becomes evident or gait impairment emerges. Parkinsonism in DIP often escapes detection in the early stages, it being diagnosed only after the patient's disease has reached a relatively advanced stage [24]. Again a characteristic feature of DIP is the symmetry of symptoms. As in drug-induced tremor, the only way to differentiate bradykinesia in DIP from that in PD is to suspend the offending drugs and observe the patient. Symptoms often resolve spontaneously within a variable time frame (from as little as one to two weeks to eight months) following withdrawal of the offending drug.

Bradykinesia in VP may vary in severity; slow-onset VP is typically bilateral and symmetrical, affecting the lower limbs more than the upper limbs (lower-body parkinsonism), and is generally considered to be characterized by a stepwise progression [25]. Patients with WD may have asymmetrical bradykinesia of varying severity but are less likely to respond to levodopa treatment than patients with typical PD [20].

Rigidity

Another cardinal feature of parkinsonism is rigidity, defined as increased resistance to passive movement of the limbs. Rigidity may be described as either cogwheel rigidity with a ratchet-like resistance, or lead pipe rigidity, having a tonic resistance throughout limb movement. The type and severity of rigidity alone are often of little help in differentiating

Table 7.5 Postural abnormalities in parkinsonism: phenomenology

PD: flexed posture of head, trunk, and limbs. Camptocormia in 5–7% of the cases

MSA: flexed posture may be accompanied by severe antecollis. Severe lateral trunk deviation (Pisa syndrome) in some cases

PSP: erect posture with retrocollis (in classical Richardson's syndrome)

CBD: lateral deviation of the trunk with fixed dystonic postures in the limbs

Vascular: variable posture. Some cases may present with a stooped posture

Wilson's disease: often asymmetrical with marked dystonic features

the various conditions with parkinsonism. Rigidity in PD is classically appendicular and asymmetrical. Cogwheel rigidity is very common in PD, and may contribute to the postural abnormalities seen in this disease [5], such as flexion of the neck, trunk, elbows, metacarpophalangeal joints, and knees (Table 7.5). When thoracolumbar spine forward flexion exceeds 45° the term camptocormia is employed. The cause of these postural abnormalities is complex and probably multifactorial, including the possible occurrence of dystonia and focal myopathic changes [26].

In patients with MSA and CBD, rigidity may be accompanied by spasticity and, particularly in the latter, by dystonic features and contractures [23,27]. The most common and specific presentation of CBD is an asymmetrical rigid dystonic jerking of the hand. Rigidity in CBD is coupled with marked difficulty in using the involved body side because of limb kinetic and ideomotor apraxia [28]. Some patients with CBD exhibit the alien limb phenomenon in which the affected limb, usually an arm, moves involuntarily, appearing to float in space without the patient's awareness [29]. Axial rigidity (primary extensor neck rigidity) is characteristic instead (although not universal) in PSP; axial rigidity confers a retrocollic appearance and is associated with less severe limb rigidity [30].

Rigidity, which is present in most patients with DIP, mainly affects the neck [24]. Increased tone in VP is usually of a mixed type (spasticity and rigidity combined) and is often associated with paratonia or *gegenhalten*. The distribution of rigidity in VP differs from that in PD insofar as it is more symmetrical in the former, mainly affecting the lower part of the body. Although rigidity in VP typically responds poorly to dopaminergic medications, some patients do experience an initial response to levodopa, which subsequently declines gradually [31]. Patients with WD typically have rigidity of the cogwheel type and exacerbated segmental tonic reflexes; these symptoms rarely respond to anti-parkinsonian drugs [20].

Balance and gait disorders

In parkinsonism, postural instability is usually combined with gait impairment. Postural instability refers to an impairment of postural-righting reflexes. In clinical practice, postural instability is assessed using the pull test, during which the examiner stands behind the patient and pulls them backwards. The response to testing is considered abnormal when patients take more than two steps to keep their balance. Although considered an integral part of PD, postural instability often appears in the later stages of the disease [4]. Patients with PSP, CBD, and MSA have prominent balance difficulties, each with additional unique features [32]. Postural instability associated with early backward falls during the first year of the disease course is a cardinal feature of classic PSP [22]. In addition, patients with PSP often have difficulty in rising from the sitting position; conversely, when sitting down, they tend to raise their feet (sitting *en bloc*). Postural instability and falls manifest themselves later in CBD than in PSP, although earlier than in PD. Unlike patients with PSP, those with CBD do not necessarily fall in one direction. Difficulty in balance is also present in MSA-P but, in contrast to PSP, recurrent falls at disease onset are relatively unusual. Patients with VP are also unsteady while standing and their balance is poor [33], whereas postural instability is a rare feature in DIP.

Another common feature of parkinsonism is gait disorder. PD patients with advanced disease typically ambulate with a stooped posture, flexed adducted arms, and loss of arm swing. Reduced arm swing during gait is often the first presenting feature of PD. Decreased height and length of step with a shuffling gait appear in the later stages of the disease. Gait in MSA is markedly affected throughout the disease course [12]; disproportionate anterocollis may frequently be seen in MSA along with severe lateral deviation of the trunk, resulting in the Pisa syndrome [34]. However, the Pisa syndrome is not peculiar to MSA; indeed, it may be seen in the late stages of PD as well as in other neurodegenerative disorders. In contrast to PD, patients with the classic PSP phenotype ambulate with an erect posture and abducted arms [22]. Another characteristic movement feature of this condition is turning *en bloc* (minimal trunk rotation while turning around).

A gait disorder is also an integral part of VP. Upper limbs are often spared, hence the term lower-body parkinsonism. The posture is upright and the base is widened, which is in contrast to the stooped posture and narrow base of PD, and there is no loss of associated movements. A gait analysis study showed that the gait in VP shares some features of cerebellar gait, and differs from the gait disturbances in PD [35]. The classic VP gait (characterized by start- and turn hesitation, short steps, a widened base, and imbalance with an inappropriate postural response) may resemble the abnormal gait of normal-pressure hydrocephalus, which represents a major differential diagnostic element for this condition. In early WD, ambulatory disturbances are observed commonly as subtle features of gait impairment; indeed, such disturbances have been described in approximately 75% of patients with the parkinsonian type of WD [20]. In the advanced stages, the combination of akinetic-rigid, ataxic, and dystonic syndromes can severely affect locomotion.

Other motor symptoms

The facial appearance of patients with parkinsonism is characterized by the gradual development of a mask-like face (hypomimia). In addition, the rate of blinking decreases, while drooling may be evident in more advanced cases. Blepharospasm may be seen in treated PD, although it is more common in PSP. The facial appearance of patients with MSA is marked by atypical spontaneous or levodopa-induced dystonia or dyskinesia, which mainly affects the orofacial muscles and occasionally resembles *risus sardonicus* [11]. A constant facial involvement is present in PSP, with a peculiar wide-eyed, non-blinking, staring expression that is more striking than the hypomimia observed in PD [36]. When patients exhibit involuntary movements of their lips during interviews, DIP should be suspected, particularly neuroleptic-induced parkinsonism. DIP may also cause a dry mouth, mainly owing to medications, which should arouse the clinician's suspicion if reported by the patients [24]. The fixed pseudo-smile or *risus sardonicus* is considered a highly characteristic facial aspect of WD, it being present in about 70% of the cases [20]. This sign, however, is not limited to WD, but has also been described in other disorders associated with basal ganglia lesions.

Speech disorders are a well-recognized complication of all parkinsonian disorders. The classic speech pattern in PD is hypokinetic dysarthria. Patients develop a soft voice with accompanying slurring. In MSA, in addition to hypokinetic speech, patients may develop ataxic and, more rarely, spastic qualities in the voice, resulting in quivery, croaky, strained, high-pitched speech [11]. Patients with PSP also have hypokinetic dysarthria, which is commonly associated with spastic elements, causing a slurred, lower pitched, growling quality of speech [22]. The characteristic moaning vocalizations in PSP are not present in any other forms of parkinsonism. Speech impairment is also frequent in CBD, with dysarthria of a mixed character (hypophonic and spastic). Unlike the dysarthria in MSA and PSP, the dysarthria in CBD often remains mild for a long period, even when general motor impairment is relatively severe. In the later stages of CBD, the peculiar characteristics of apraxic speech (slow speaking rate, abnormal prosody, and distorted sound substitutions, repetitions, and prolongations) in association with signs of non-fluent aphasia may help in the differential diagnosis. In VP, dysarthria may be associated with dysphagia and emotional lability, which are common components of pseudobulbar palsy. Hence, although the early development of severe dysarthria may be suggestive of AP, it cannot reliably be used to distinguish between conditions such as MSA, PSP, CBD, and VP. Dysarthria is also a frequent neurological manifestation in patients with WD [20,37] and is characterized by several speech abnormalities, including lower volume, hoarseness, difficulty in initiating speech, and altered intonation. If the disease is not treated, the dysarthria worsens leading to complete anarthria.

Parkinsonism is also associated with a wide range of altered eye movements. Impaired vision with insufficient convergence or altered pursuit and saccades may occur in PD, PSP, MSA, and CBD. Although oculomotor dysfunction may develop only years after the initial symptoms in PSP, it is of major diagnostic value. Classically, PSP causes impairment in vertical saccadic movement associated with a decreased horizontal saccadic velocity. A marked slowing in vertical saccadic movement precedes the development of vertical supranuclear palsy. Supranuclear gaze palsy initially affects downgaze (upgaze impairment is a common change that may occur as a result of aging, and is thus of no diagnostic value), but may later spread to ocular movements in the horizontal plane. Evidence that oculomotor disorders are supranuclear in origin comes from the dissociation between impaired voluntary movements and pursuit gaze and the preservation of oculocephalic reflexes. The impairment of downward opticokinetic nystagmus may also help distinguish PSP from PD [38]. Other oculomotor abnormalities in PSP include square wave jerks (which are uncommon in PD), convergence insufficiency, reduced blink rate, eyelid apraxia (difficulty in opening or closing eyelids) accompanied by compensatory eyebrow elevation, with overactivity of the frontalis and procerus muscles, and blepharospasm [39]. Oculomotor abnormalities, particularly problems in looking downward, can make simple tasks such as eating and descending stairs difficult. In contrast to PSP, which is associated with markedly decreased saccadic velocity, in CBD saccadic velocity is relatively preserved [39]. Some patients with CBD, nevertheless, have oculomotor impairments that resemble those observed in PSP. Other associated oculomotor abnormalities in CBD are oculomotor apraxia, optic ataxia, and simultanagnosia [40]. In MSA, oculomotor abnormalities may include square wave jerks (owing to fixation instability), ocular dysmetria, which may include hypometric or hypermetric saccades or both, although with normal velocity and latency, as well as nystagmus [11]. Lastly, oculomotor abnormalities have been described regularly in WD. These include nystagmus, conjugate ocular palsy, saccadic alterations, and oculogyric crises [41,42]. The Kayser–Fleischer ring, owing to copper deposition in Descemet's membrane in the cornea, is an important ocular sign found in virtually all neurological cases of WD.

Non-motor symptoms

All parkinsonian patients have a variety of non-motor symptoms that not only may significantly affect patient's quality of life but are also key elements in discriminating these diseases.

Olfactory abnormalities

Olfactory dysfunction (hyposmia) is a frequent (80–100%) and early abnormality in PD [43]. Olfactory loss could be the earliest sign in PD, manifesting even at a preclinical motor stage [44]. Although most reports show little or no correlation with disease duration [45,46], others have suggested that hyposmia correlates with motor disability [47]. Whether these findings represent a true progression in olfactory function, or are partly related to an impairment in the ability to sniff is unclear [48]. In contrast to patients with PD, patients with MSA have a preserved sense of smell or only a mild smell deficit [49,50]. Conversely, in PSP and CBD, olfactory function is normal [51,52]. Evidence that olfactory function in VP does not differ from that in controls suggests that olfactory evaluation could have a useful role in the differential diagnosis between PD and VP [53]. A study investigating patients with DIP reported that in some of those with hyposmia who failed to recover after discontinuing the therapy, olfactory function remained abnormal [54]. This finding suggests that some patients with presumed DIP could have underlying PD that is unmasked by neuroleptics. However, it should be considered that many patients with DIP are affected by chronic psychosis that is also associated with olfactory impairment. Patients with the neurological variant of WD also have more severe olfactory dysfunction than patients with the hepatic type; individuals who are more severely affected present with a more pronounced olfactory deficit [55].

Sleep abnormalities

Nearly all patients with PD have some form of sleep disruption and this problem usually starts early in the disease course [56]. About 30% of male patients (women are less affected) with PD experience rapid eye movement (REM) sleep behavior disorder (RBD). This event, a form of parasomnia characterized by loss of the normal skeletal muscle atonia during REM sleep, enables patients to physically enact their dreams, which are often vivid or unpleasant [57]. Partners commonly report vocalizations (shouting, talking) and abnormal movements (arm or leg jerks, violent assault, falling out of bed). Like olfactory disturbances, RBD might precede the development of motor signs in PD. Excessive daytime sleepiness (EDS) and involuntary dozing affect up to 50% of PD patients and could also be a preclinical marker [58]. EDS is probably a result of a combination of a disease process, the effect of nocturnal sleep disruption, and the use of anti-parkinsonian drugs. In some patients with parkinsonism, EDS is linked to the development of sudden-onset sleep, which is potentially dangerous if the individuals drive. RBD is also present in patients with MSA [59] and isolated RBD has been suggested as a possible early symptom of this disease, before any motor symptom. RBD and other sleep disorders are more common in patients with MSA than in those with PD, matched for disease duration. Patients with MSA also have nocturnal inspiratory stridor and obstructive sleep apnoea that can cause sudden death [59]. These symptoms are among the common symptoms at onset and tend to be associated with more severe motor function impairment. Sleep disturbances (insomnia, shorter sleep latency, and increased number of awakenings) are less evident in PSP [60]. In conclusion, RBD is a disorder frequently associated with PD and MSA, and much more rarely with PSP [61]. The sleep pattern of patients with WD is characterized by a larger number of nocturnal awakenings, which correlate to nightmares and palpitations [62]. Patients with WD complain of not feeling rested after sleep, needing frequent daytime naps, and becoming fatigued during the day. Some patients with WD also experience sleep paralysis and cataplexy.

Autonomic failure

Autonomic dysfunction is a key characteristic of MSA and occurs with varying severity in PD and in other syndromes with parkinsonism. Many patients with parkinsonism complain of a generic respiratory dysfunction with shortness of breath, sometimes owing to underlying cardiac or pulmonary disease, or an accompanying restrictive lung pattern, presumably arising from chest wall and diaphragmatic rigidity and overall bradykinesia. Respiratory dysfunction is often associated with sleep disturbances, particularly in patients with MSA.

In the past decade, an increasing relationship has emerged between many conditions with parkinsonism and cardiovascular autonomic dysfunction. The most important cardiovascular alteration in parkinsonism is orthostatic hypotension (OH), commonly seen late in the course of PD [63]. The diagnosis of OH requires an orthostatic fall in systolic blood pressure of more than 20 mmHg or a fall in diastolic pressure of more than 10 mmHg [64]. Although some studies reported OH in the early stages of PD, an early finding of OH in a patient with parkinsonism is more likely to suggest a diagnosis of MSA [65]. Because of compensatory changes in cerebral blood flow autoregulation, patients who have MSA may remain initially asymptomatic despite large decreases in systolic and diastolic blood pressure. In patients with symptomatic OH, this may manifest with neck and shoulder ache and changes in visual perception, later leading to orthostatic syncope and even sudden death [65]. Anti-parkinsonian treatments usually worsen OH. In addition to OH, patients with MSA have decreased heart rate variability during forced respiration [66]. Other conditions with parkinsonism such as PSP and CBD can also manifest some signs of OH, but not with the prevalence and degree as in MSA [66].

Gastrointestinal dysfunction is another common manifestation of parkinsonism [32]. Constipation is one of the most frequent non-motor symptoms in PD and, according to some epidemiological studies, might even precede the development of the motor disorder by several years. During disease progression constipation may severely impair patients' quality of life. Patients with MSA also manifest a variety of gastrointestinal problems [67]. Earlier manifestation of swallowing difficulties suggests AP, because in PD severe swallowing problems are present only late in the disease course. Prominent dysphagia is a characteristic of PSP and MSA. Patients with PSP persistently overfill their mouths when eating, owing to severe frontal lobe involvement. Dysphagia is a manifestation of VP as a part of pseudobulbar palsy [68]. In WD, dysphagia is a universal problem and occasionally develops into a severe swallowing disorder, needing enteral alimentation by feeding tube; drooling is frequently associated [20].

Genitourinary dysfunction should alert the clinician to a possible diagnosis of AP, even if the frequent confounding problem of prostate enlargement in elderly men should always be taken into account. Bladder dysfunction differs in PD and MSA [67]. Although frequency and urgency of micturition are common in both disorders, notable urge or stress incontinence

Table 7.6 Genitourinary disorders in parkinsonism

Urinary dysfunction	PD	MSA	PSP	DLB	HD
Polyuria	+(+)	++	+	+(+)	+
Urgency	+(+)	++	+	+(+)	
Incontinence	++ (late)	+++	+	++	+
Nocturia	+(+)	++	+	+(+)	+
Difficulties in initiating micturition	+(+)	++	+	+(+)	+
Chronic retention	+ (late)	+++	+	++	+
Sexual dysfunction					
Erectile dysfunction	++ (late)	+++	+	++	+
Loss of ejaculation	++ (late)	++	?	++	+

Frequency of each symptom was rated increasingly from + to +++

with continuous leakage is not a feature of PD, and when present these symptoms manifest only in advanced disease (Table 7.6). Common complaints in PD are urgency and increased daytime frequency and difficulty in initiating micturition. Night-time frequency is among the most troublesome urinary complaints of advanced PD [69]. Conversely, early urinary incontinence consisting of involuntary partial or total bladder emptying is a typical characteristic of patients with MSA [65]. Sexual dysfunction in PD could be a component of dysautonomia, and some reports describe both reduced and abnormally increased sex interest or desire [70]. In contrast, erectile dysfunction is an early and universal symptom, often accompanying bladder dysfunction, in men with MSA [71]: it has also been suggested that it may appear even five to ten years before the motor symptoms of this disease. Although sexual function may deteriorate in women with MSA, little is known about this feature of MSA [72]. PSP can also manifest with urological dysfunction early in its course, but the symptom is less specific diagnostically in PSP than in MSA.

Skin problems are another manifestation of autonomic dysfunction in parkinsonism. PD is commonly associated with seborrhoea, dermatitis, eczema, and spontaneous or iatrogenic edema. Leg edema in PD has multiple causes and is frequently asymmetrical with greater severity on the initial side of the body affected by the parkinsonism. Compared with patients with PD, patients with MSA more often have profound spontaneous edema: they may also have cold, violaceous-appearing hands or feet, with poor circulatory return after blanching by pressure [11]. Many patients with MSA also report cold sensitivity or Raynaud's phenomena [11,73]. There is no available information about skin changes in other examples of AP.

Sensory abnormalities

Among the non-motor manifestations of parkinsonism are sensory disturbances. The most common sensory symptom reported by patients with early PD is shoulder pain. In more advanced cases, pain may be related to motor fluctuations (early morning dystonia), or a result of secondary causes such as musculoskeletal problems [74]. Another type of pain described in PD is a deep visceral, oral, and genital pain [75,76]. Sensory dysfunction is the hallmark of patients with CBD and includes cortical sensory deficits and alien limb phenomenon [77,78]. Although patients with PSP may have limb apraxia, it is less severe in PSP than in CBD [79]. Different types of sensory loss and pain are described in VP, reflecting the location of the cerebral vascular lesion [80].

Cognitive and behavioral disorders

All forms of parkinsonism lead to some degree of cognitive and behavioral impairment related to changes in several brain neurotransmitters including dopamine, noradrenaline, serotonin, and acetylcholine. Anxiety and depression are common in PD and may manifest before the onset of its motor symptoms [81]; anxiety can present as panic attacks, phobias, or generalized anxiety disorder, and in patients with motor fluctuations anxiety is often evident during motor blocks. Depression can be present in the majority of patients with PD and is characterized by apathy (loss of volition), feeling of guilt, lack of self-esteem, and sadness [82]. Mood symptoms such as anxiety, depression, emotional lability, and apathy are also particularly common in VP [83]. In contrast to PD and VP, patients with PSP have more changes in insight, disinhibition, and apathy than true depression [84,85]. These changes often become apparent at an early disease stage.

Major cognitive changes are unusual in early PD and their presence points toward another condition. Some studies suggest that the various examples of AP may be distinguished from differences in executive function [86]. For example, PSP and CBD cause profound cognitive difficulties whereas MSA leads only to executive dysfunction (similar to that typically seen during early PD). By definition, in dementia with Lewy bodies (DLB) cognitive decline precedes the onset of parkinsonism or in some cases follows it very shortly. Patients with PD, in whom dementia develops more than 12 months after the initial motor symptoms, should be diagnosed as PD with dementia rather than with DLB [87]. Psychological and behavioral problems are also typical of DLB. Both problems can be among the first manifestations of DLB, even preceding substantial cognitive decline. A specific characteristic of DLB is fluctuating cognition and attention: these changes interfere with cognitive assessment and lead to high variability in cognitive performances [88]. Disproportionate early visuospatial deficits and visuoconstructional dysfunction are other useful diagnostic indicators for DLB [89,90]. Psychotic symptoms can also manifest early in the course of DLB, consisting of spontaneous recurrent visual hallucinations and delusional misidentifications, which are present in two-thirds of these patients [91]. In contrast to DLB, hallucinations in PD develop later in the disease course and are frequently induced by concurrent infection, dehydration, or use of high doses of dopaminergic drugs. Like the visual hallucinations in DLB, hallucinations in PD have a complex form, rich in details and color, involving human figures and animals. Emotional responses to this experience vary from complete indifference to intense fear. Because CBD affects the parietal lobe, it typically manifests with cognitive and behavioral symptoms caused by cortical involvement. The hallmarks of CBD, alien limb, cortical sensory loss, and limb kinetic and ideomotor apraxia, are never seen in PD. Hemispatial neglect can be a common feature, along with disinhibition and dysphasia [92]. Signs of pseudobulbar palsy, such as crying or laughing spells or both, may become evident in many conditions with parkinsonism including MSA, PSP, VP, and rarely PD [53]. Psychiatric manifestations are universal and varied in WD [41]. The most frequent are depression, emotional lability, irritability, and disinhibition, but some patients also have more severe psychiatric symptoms including catatonia, agitation, aggressiveness, delusional thoughts, and mania.

Future perspectives

The diagnosis of the various forms of parkinsonism still relies on an accurate examination of the patient and on the clinical skills of the examiner. The use of ancillary tests (MRI, SPECT and PET, transcranial Doppler sonography, cardiovascular autonomic testing, neurophysiological investigations) may help the diagnostic work-up of patients with parkinsonism, but at present the results from investigations are rarely specific and their cost effectiveness remains to be established. A possible exception is positive genetic testing, which allows the confirmation of some uncommon forms of parkinsonism (monogenic autosomal dominant or recessive PD, Westphal variant of Huntington's disease, pantothenate kinase-associated neurodegeneration). A final consideration is that in making the correct clinical diagnosis of patients with parkinsonism, it is important to be prepared to modify the diagnosis whenever new features appear, suggesting a different condition than the one initially suspected.

References

1. Litvan I, Bhatia KP, Burn DJ, et al. Movement Disorders Society Scientific Issues Committee report: SIC Task Force appraisal of clinical diagnostic criteria for Parkinsonian disorders. *Mov Disord* 2003; **18**: 467–86.

2. Hughes AJ, Daniel SE, Ben-Shlomo Y, et al. The accuracy of diagnosis of parkinsonian syndromes in a specialist movement disorder service. *Brain* 2002; **125**: 861–70.

3. Katzenschlager R, Cardozo A, Avila Cobo MA, et al. Unclassifiable parkinsonism in two European tertiary referral centres for movement disorders. *Mov Disord* 2003; **18**: 1123–31.

4. Hoehn MM, Yahr MD. Parkinsonism: onset, progression and mortality. *Neurology* 1967; **17**: 427–42.

5. Poewe WH, Wenning GK. The natural history of PD. *Ann Neurol* 1998; **44**: S1–9.

6. Hughes AJ, Daniel SE, Blankson S, et al. A clinicopathologic study of 100 cases of Parkinson's disease. *Arch Neurol* 1993; **50**: 140–8.

7. Deuschl G, Bain P, Brin M. Consensus statement of the Movement Disorder Society on Tremor. Ad Hoc Scientific Committee. *Mov Disord* 1998; **13**: 2–23.

8. Hunker CJ, Abbs JH. Uniform frequency of parkinsonian resting tremor in the lips, jaw, tongue, and index finger. *Mov Disord* 1990; **5**: 71–7.

9. Verghese J, Lipton RB, Dickson DW, et al. A clinicopathological study of rest tremors in the elderly. *J Am Geriatr Soc* 2004; **52**: 1781–3.

10. Meara J, Bhowmick BK, Hobson P. Accuracy of diagnosis in patients with presumed Parkinson's disease. *Age Ageing* 1999; **28**: 99–102.

11. Quinn NP. How to diagnose multiple system atrophy. *Mov Disord* 2005; **20**: S5–10.

12. Wenning GK, Shlomo IB, Magalhaes M, et al. Clinical features and natural history of multiple system atrophy. *Brain* 1994; **117**: 835–45.

13. Colosimo C, Albanese A, Hughes AJ, et al. Some specific clinical features differentiate multiple system atrophy (striatonigral variety) from Parkinson's disease. *Arch Neurol* 1995; **52**: 294–8.

14. Williams DR, De Silva R, Paviour DC, et al. Characteristics of two distinct clinical phenotypes in pathologically proven progressive supranuclear palsy: Richardson's syndrome and PSP-parkinsonism. *Brain* 2005; **128**: 1247–58.

15. Kompoliti K, Goetz CG, Boeve BF, et al. Clinical presentation and pharmacological therapy in corticobasal degeneration. *Arch Neurol* 1998; **55**: 957–61.

16. Bower JH, Maraganore DM, McDonnell SK, et al. Incidence and distribution of parkinsonism in Olmsted County; Minnesota, 1976–1990. *Neurology* 1999; **52**: 1214–20.

17. Critchley M. Arteriosclerotic parkinsonism. *Brain* 1929; **52**: 23–83.

18. Bower JH, Dickson DW, Taylor L, et al. Clinical correlates of the pathology

underlying parkinsonism: a population perspective. *Mov Disord* 2002; **17**: 910–16.

19. Miwa H, Hatori K, Kondon T, et al. Thalamic tremor: case reports and implications of the tremor-generating mechanisms. *Neurology* 1996; **46**: 75–9.

20. Machado A, Chien HF, Deguti MM, et al. Neurological manifestations in Wilson's disease. *Mov Disord* 2006; **21**: 2192–6.

21. Matsuo H, Takashima H, Kishikawa M, et al. Pure akinesia: an atypical manifestation of progressive supranuclear palsy. *J Neurol Neurosurg Psychiatry* 1991; **54**: 397–400.

22. Litvan I, Campbell G, Mangone CA, et al. Which clinical features differentiate progressive supranuclear palsy from related disorders? A clinicopathological study. *Brain* 1997; **120**: 65–74.

23. Stover NP, Watts RL. Corticobasal degeneration. *Semin Neurol* 2001; **21**: 49–58.

24. Chou KL, Friedman JH. Drug-induced parkinsonism in the elderly. *Future Neurol* 2007; **2**: 307–16.

25. Demirkiran M, Bozdemir H, Sarica Y. Vascular parkinsonism: a distinct, heterogeneous clinical entity. *Acta Neurol Scand* 2001; **104**: 63–7.

26. Schabitz WR, Glatz K, Schuhan C, et al. Severe forward flexion of the trunk in Parkinson's disease: focal myopathy of the paraspinal muscles mimicking camptocormia. *Mov Disord* 2003; **18**: 408–14.

27. Gouider-Khouja N, Vidaihet M, Bonnet AM, et al. Pure striatonigral degeneration and Parkinson's disease: a comparative clinical study. *Mov Disord* 1995; **10**: 288–94.

28. Zodikoff C, Lang AE. Apraxia in movement disorders. *Brain* 2005; **128**: 1480–97.

29. Doody RS, Jankovic J. The alien hand and related sign. *J Neurol Neurosurg Psychiatry* 1999; **55** : 806–10.

30. Collins SJ, Ahlskog JE, Parisi JE, et al. Progressive supranuclear palsy: neuropathologically based diagnostic clinical criteria. *J Neurol Neurosurg Psychiatry* 1995; **58**: 167–73.

31. Mark MH, Sage JI, Walters AS, et al. Binswanger disease presenting as levodopa-responsive parkinsonism: clinicopathologic study of three cases. *Mov Disord* 1995; **10**: 450–4.

32. Tuite PJ, Krawczewski K. Parkinsonism: A review-of-systems approach to diagnosis. *Semin Neurol* 2007; **27**: 113–22.

33. Zijlmans JCM, Poels PJE, van der Straaten, et al. Quantitative gait analysis in patients with vascular parkinsonism. *Mov Disord* 1996; **11**: 501–8.

34. Colosimo C. Pisa syndrome in a patient with multiple system atrophy. *Mov Disord* 1998; **13**: 607–9.

35. Ebersbach G, Sojet M, Valldeoriola F, et al. Comparative analysis of gait in Parkinson's disease, cerebellar ataxia and subcortical arteriosclerotic encephalopathy. *Brain* 1999; **122**: 1349–55.

36. Romano S, Colosimo C. Procerus sign in progressive supranuclear palsy. *Neurology* 2001; **57**: 1928.

37. Stremmel W, Meyerrose KW, Niederau C, et al. Wilson's disease: clinical presentation, treatment, and survival. *Ann Intern Med* 1991; **115**: 720–6.

38. Garbutt S, Riley DE, Kumar AN, et al. Abnormalities of optokinetic nystagmus in progressive supranuclear palsy. *J Neurol Neurosurg Psychiatry* 2004; **75**: 1386–94.

39. Rivaud-Pechoux S, Vidailhet M, Gallouedec G, et al. Longitudinal ocular motor study in corticobasal degeneration and progressive supranuclear palsy. *Neurology* 2000; **54**: 1029–32.

40. Mendez MF. Corticobasal ganglionic degeneration with Balint's syndrome. *J Neuropsych Clin Neurosci* 2000; **12**: 273–5.

41. Hoogenraad T. Clinical manifestation. In: Hoogenraad T, ed. *Wilson's disease*. London: WB Saunders, 1996; 71–108.

42. Lee MS, Kim YD, Lyoo CH. Oculogyric crisis as an initial manifestation of Wilson's disease. *Neurology* 1999; **52**: 1714–5.

43. Katzenschlager R, Lees A. Olfaction and Parkinson's syndromes: its role in differential diagnosis. *Curr Opin Neurol* 2004; **17**: 417–23.

44. Markopoulou K, Larsen KW, Wszolek EK, et al. Olfactory dysfunction in familial parkinsonism. *Neurology* 1997; **49**: 1262–7.

45. Hawkes CH, Shephard BC. Olfactory evoked responses and identification tests in neurological disease. *Ann NY Acad Sci* 1998; **855**: 608–15.

46. Doty RL, Deems DA, Stellar S. Olfactory dysfunction in parkinsonism: a general deficit unrelated to neurologic signs, disease stage or disease duration. *Neurology* 1988; **38**: 1237–44.

47. Tissingh G, Berendse HW, Bergmans P, et al. Loss of olfaction in de novo and treated Parkinson's disease: possible implications for early diagnosis. *Mov Disord* 2001; **16**: 41–6.

48. Sobel N, Prabhakaran V, Hartley CA, et al. Odorant-induced and sniff-induced activation in the cerebellum of the human. *J Neurosci* 1998; **18**: 8990–9001.

49. Wenning GK, Shephard B, Magalhaes M, et al. Olfactory function in multiple system atrophy. *Neurodegeneration* 1993; **2**: 169–71.

50. Abele M, Riet A, Hummel T, et al. Olfactory dysfunction in cerebellar ataxia and multiple system atrophy. *J Neurol* 2003; **250**: 1453–5.

51. Wenning GK, Shephard B, Hawkes C, et al. Olfactory function in progressive supranuclear palsy and corticobasal degeneration. *J Neurol Neurosurg Psychiatry* 1995; **57**: 251–2.

52. Doty RL, Golbe LI, McKeown DA, et al. Olfactory testing differentiates between progressive supranuclear palsy and idiopathic Parkinson's disease. *Neurology* 1993; **43**: 962–5.

53. Winikates J, Jankovic J. Clinical correlates of vascular parkinsonism. *Arch Neurol* 1999; **56**: 98–102.

54. Hensiek AE, Bhatia K, Hawkes CH. Olfactory function in drug-induced parkinsonism. *J Neurol* 2000; **247**: P303.

55. Mueller A, Reuner U, Landis B, et al. Extrapyramidal symptoms in Wilson's disease are associated with olfactory dysfunction. *Mov Disord* 2006; **21**: 1311–16.

56. Chaudhuri KR. Nocturnal symptoms complex in PD and its management. *Neurology* 2003; **61**: S17–23.

57. Cagnon JF, Bedard MA, Fantini ML, et al. REM sleep behaviour disorder and REM sleep without atonia in Parkinson's disease. *Neurology* 2002; **59**: 585–9.

58. Abbott RD, Ross GW, White LR, et al. Excessive daytime sleepiness and the future risk of Parkinson's disease. *Mov Disord* 2005; **20**: S101.

59. Ghorayeb I, Bioulac B, Tison F. Sleep disorders in multiple system atrophy. *J Neural Transm* 2005; **112**: 1669–75.

60. Aldrich MS, Foster NL, White RF, et al. Sleep abnormalities in progressive supranuclear palsy. *Ann Neurol* 1989; **25**: 577–81.

61. Boeve BF, Silber MH, Ferman TJ, et al. Association of REM sleep behaviour disorder and neurodegenerative disease may reflect an underlying synucleinopathy. *Mov Disord* 2001; **16**: 622–30.

62. Portala K, Westermark K, Ekselius L, et al. Sleep in patients with treated Wilson's disease. A questionnaire study. *Nord J Psychiatry* 2002; **56**: 291–7.

63. Goldstein DS. Dysautonomia in Parkinson's disease: neurocardiological abnormalities. *Lancet Neurol* 2003; **2**: 669–76.

64. Consensus statement on the definition of orthostatic hypotension, pure autonomic failure, and multiple system atrophy. The Consensus Committee of the American Autonomic Society and the American Academy of Neurology. *Neurology* 1996; **46**: 1470.

65. Gilman S, Low PA, Quinn N, et al. Consensus statement on the diagnosis of multiple system atrophy. *J Neurol Sci* 1999; **163**: 94–8.

66. Holmberg B, Kallio M, Johnels B, et al. Cardiovascular reflex testing contributes to clinical evaluation and differential diagnosis of parkinsonian syndromes. *Mov Disord* 2001; **16**: 217–25.

67. Wenning GK, Colosimo C, Geser F, et al. Multiple system atrophy. *Lancet Neurol* 2004; **3**: 93–103.

68. Sibon I, Tison F. Vascular parkinsonism. *Curr Opin Neurol* 2004; **17**: 49–54.

69. Sakakibara R, Shinotoh H, Uchiyama T, et al. Questionnaire-based assessment of pelvic organ dysfunction in Parkinson's disease. *Auton Neurosci* 2001; **92**: 76–85.

70. Brown RG, Jahanshahi M, Quinn N, et al. Sexual function in patients with Parkinson's disease and their partners. *J Neurol Neurosurg Psychiatry* 1990; **12**: 480–6.

71. Kirchhof K, Apostolidis AN, Mathias CJ, et al. Erectile and urinary dysfunction may be the presenting features in patients with multiple system atrophy: a retrospective study. *Int J Impot Res* 2003; **15**: 293–8.

72. Oertel WH, Wachter T, Quinn NP, et al. Reduced genital sensitivity in female patients with multiple system atrophy of parkinsonian type. *Mov Disord* 2003;**18**: 430–2.

73. Colosimo C, Geser F, Benarroch EE, et al. Multiple system atrophy. In: Gilman S, ed. *Neurobiology of disease*. San Diego (CA): Academic Press, 2007; 83–93.

74. Quinn N, Koller WC, Lang AE, et al. Painful Parkinson's disease. *Lancet* 1996; **1**: 1366–9.

75. Chaudhuri KR, Healy DG, Schapira A. Non-motor symptoms of Parkinson's disease: diagnosis and management. *Lancet Neurol* 2006; **5**: 235–45.

76. Ford B, Louise P, Greene P, et al. Oral and genital pain syndromes in Parkinson's disease. *Mov Disord* 1996; **11**: 421–6.

77. Bhatia KP, Lang AE. Corticobasal degeneration. In: Flint Beal M, Lang AE, Ludolph A, eds. *Neurodegenerative diseases*. Cambridge: Cambridge University Press, 2005; 682–96.

78. Belfor N, Amici S, Boxer AL, et al. Clinical and neuropsychological features of corticobasal degeneration. *Mech Ageing and Dev* 2006; **127**: 203–7.

79. Pharr V, Uttl B, Stark M, et al. Comparison of apraxia in corticobasal degeneration and progressive supranuclear palsy. *Neurology* 2001; **56**: 957–63.

80. Rektor I, Rektorova I, Kubova D. Vascular parkinsonism – an update. *J Neurol Sci* 2006; **248**: 185–91.

81. Shiba M, Bower JH, Maraganore DM, et al. Anxiety disorders and depressive disorders preceding Parkinson's disease: a case-control study. *Mov Disord* 2000; **15**: 669–77.

82. Burn DJ. Beyond the iron mask: towards better recognition and treatment of depression associated with Parkinson's disease. *Mov Disord* 2002; **17**: 445–54.

83. O'Brien JT, Erkinjuntti T, Reisberg B, et al. Vascular cognitive impairment. *Lancet Neurol* 2003; **2** : 89–98.

84. Aarsland D, Litvan I, Larsen JP. Neuropsychiatric symptoms of patients with progressive supranuclear palsy and Parkinson's disease. *J Neuropsychiatry Clin Neurosci* 2001; **13**: 42–9.

85. Burn DJ, Lees AJ. Progressive supranuclear palsy: where are we now? *Lancet Neurol* 2001; **1**: 359–69.

86. Lange KW, Tucha O, Alders GL, et al. Differentiation of parkinsonian syndromes according to differences in executive functions. *J Neural Transm* 2003; **110**: 983–95.

87. McKeith IG, Galasko D, Kosava K, et al. Consensus guidelines for the clinical and pathologic diagnosis of dementia with Lewy bodies: report of the consortium on DLB international workshop. *Neurology* 1996; **47**: 1113–24.

88. Lambon RMA, Powell J, Howard D, et al. Semantic memory is impaired in both dementia with Lewy bodies and dementia of Alzheimer type: a comparative neuropsychological study and literature review. *J Neurol Neurosurg Psychiatry* 2001; **70**: 149–56.

89. Granalingham KK, Byrne EJ, Thornton A. Clock-face drawing to differentiate Lewy body and Alzheimer type dementia syndromes. *Lancet* 1996; **347**: 696–7.

90. Noe E, Marder K, Bell KL, et al. Comparison of dementia with Lewy bodies to Alzheimer's disease and Parkinson's disease with dementia. *Mov Disord* 2004; **19**: 60–7.

91. Ballard C, Holmes C, McKeith I, et al. Psychiatric morbidity in dementia with Lewy bodies: a prospective clinical and neuropathological comparative study with Alzheimer disease. *Am J Psychiatry* 1999; **156**: 1039–45.

92. Graham NL, Bak T, Patterson K, et al. Language function and dysfunction in corticobasal degeneration. *Neurology* 2003; **61**: 493–9.

Non-pharmacological treatment for atypical parkinsonism

Johanna G. Kalf, Marten Munneke, Bastiaan R. Bloem

Introduction

Patients who have been diagnosed with a form of atypical parkinsonism (AP) usually face a very poor prognosis. Disease progression is typically more rapid compared to Parkinson's disease (PD). Moreover, many complications that eventually occur in PD will generally develop in a much earlier phase of the disease for patients with AP and also tend to be more pronounced. One generic pattern that applies to nearly all forms of AP relates to gait impairment and postural instability [1]. Most patients with AP will experience marked walking problems or difficulties maintaining balance in the first few years of their disease. Repeated falls and injuries can occur even within the first 12 months after onset of the first symptoms, and this would be highly unusual for patients with PD. Loss of independence develops much earlier for patients with AP, and many patients can eventually move only with much assistance or become completely immobilized (the "wheelchair sign"). For example, development of postural instability and recurrent falls early in the course of the disease is an important feature that helps to distinguish progressive supranuclear palsy (PSP) from PD [2,3]. Other symptoms that are almost universally present in an early and severe form in AP include speech and swallowing disorders, and marked problems with manual dexterity, causing severe problems with activities of daily living. A more specific illustration is autonomic dysfunction, which can be present early in the course of multiple system atrophy (MSA).

The problems of patients with AP are compounded by the fact that most symptoms and signs respond poorly (if at all) to dopaminergic treatment. Stereotactic surgery is usually no option for patients with AP. Even with optimal medical management using drugs or neurosurgery, patients with AP are faced with progressively increasing impairments (for example, in speech or movement-related functions), activity limitations (self-care and mobility, for example), and restrictions in participation (as in domestic life and social activities). In fact, pharmacotherapy can sometimes worsen the situation; for instance, when dopaminergic medication aggravates orthostatic hypotension in patients with MSA. This is precisely why allied healthcare and other forms of non-pharmacological treatment are such an important cornerstone in the management of patients with AP [4,5]. Indeed, it is felt that for many patients, allied health interventions can be regarded as their primary treatment option [6], supporting patients to deal individually with the sequelae of their disease.

Non-pharmacological treatment includes physical therapy, occupational therapy, and speech–language therapy, as well as help delivered by dieticians, social workers, or sexologists. Allied healthcare has long been regarded as being much of an art, based on poorly

Handbook of Atypical Parkinsonism, eds. Carlo Colosimo, David E. Riley, and Gregor K. Wenning. Published by Cambridge University Press. © Cambridge University Press 2011.

described know-how passed on by teachers and supplemented with personal experience. However, allied healthcare is rapidly maturing as an evidence-based profession. Indeed, physical therapists, occupational therapists, and speech–language therapists can now base their clinical decisions increasingly on evidence-based guidelines that have been developed in recent years [7–10], which are described further in this chapter.

Generic principles of allied healthcare

For an optimal effect of allied healthcare interventions in patients with parkinsonism, some general treatment principles have to be considered [11] (Table 8.1). The site where treatment is delivered is an important factor to consider. Delivering the treatment in the therapist's office or a rehabilitation setting can be attractive, not only to reduce the travel time for therapists, but also because specific equipment is sometimes required. For example, exercise training can be done safely in a specific training facility with close supervision by expert personnel. A rehabilitation setting can also be useful when patients require concurrent treatment by multiple therapists, which is often the case for patients with AP. However, many limitations in participation and daily activities are often related to the patient's specific home environment. For example, freezing of gait may be suppressed when patients are tested in the therapist's office, but it can take dramatic forms when patients are observed in their own homes. The risk of falling can only be monitored properly at home, where poor lighting, loose rugs on the floor, and tight quarters in crammed living rooms markedly increase the likelihood of falling. Therefore, promoting and supporting many everyday activities take place preferably at home [12], perhaps interspersed with dedicated therapeutic sessions in the therapist's office.

Involving the caregiver is usually necessary, especially when cognitive functioning of the patient has declined. Caregivers are not supposed to fulfill the role of therapists, but can learn to assist the patient in using cues or cognitive movement strategies, for example. This becomes especially important when patients develop depression or apathy. The caregiver can

Table 8.1 Generic principles of allied healthcare

Treatment can be delivered at several sites

- therapist's office
- rehabilitation centre
- at home
- combinations

Involvement of the caregiver is vital

Treatment programs are individually adjusted, considering

- physical abilities
- cognitive abilities
- energy level
- depression and apathy

Individual versus group treatment

Safety issues

Financial issues

assist in making the necessary home adjustments, as some patients are reluctant to implement these adaptations.

Patients with parkinsonism are usually treated individually. This has the obvious advantage that the nature and intensity of any treatment program can be adjusted to each patient's specific abilities, both physically and cognitively. The energy level is also important, because some treatment programs can be fairly intensive (for example, dysarthria treatment that usually requires a series of frequent therapeutic sessions). Group treatment would be more cost effective because one therapist can train multiple patients simultaneously. Training along with other patients also creates peer pressure that may promote treatment compliance. However, most interventions ask for individual and precise feedback, so group treatment remains useful mainly as a supplemental option.

Safety is another important issue. Promoting mobility and increasing overall physical activity levels have obvious advantages, but also increase the risk of sustaining falls or injuries. This is particularly true for patients with cognitive impairment, who may fail to appreciate the risks of walking or swallowing. For example, patients with PSP have an unusually high risk of sustaining fall-related injuries. This is caused not only because PSP patients have prominent and rapidly progressive postural instability, but also because they display motor recklessness: many patients with PSP move abruptly and seem unable to judge the risk of their actions properly. The same motor recklessness also underlies the high incidence of car accidents in this disorder. Therefore, it may be necessary to supervise the patient's activities, again underscoring the need to involve the caregivers. The case is not closed whether it is ethically and morally justified to restrict a patient's activities markedly when the risks of complications are high (for example, tying patients with wandering behavior, and a high risk of falling, to a bed).

Finally, depending on specific national or perhaps even local circumstances, financial issues may pose barriers that hamper a more widespread use of allied healthcare. Patients or even physicians may feel reluctant to consider a referral to allied healthcare when treatment is not or is only partially reimbursed.

Challenges for allied healthcare in atypical parkinsonism

Prescribing allied healthcare to patients with AP comes with several specific challenges (Table 8.2). The existing evidence is based almost exclusively on studies performed in patients with PD. Indeed, even the available clinical expertise and expert opinion remains limited for patients with AP, simply because these disorders are much less common. Consequently, most descriptions and recommendations made in this chapter are based on guidelines developed primarily for PD, supplemented with limited evidence from studies in patients with AP and expert opinion.

A further concern relates to the disease pathology, which is typically much more widespread in the nervous system of patients with AP. First, the presence of lesions outside the basal ganglia circuitries may have consequences for the effectiveness of allied health treatment in AP. When treating PD patients, allied health therapists typically exploit the possibility of bypassing the defective basal ganglia by engaging intact cortical pathways and sensory systems. For example, consciously making larger strides when walking or phonating louder when talking is a relatively easy method for mildly to moderately affected PD patients to overcome their hypokinesia. Similarly, use of guided visual feedback can assist patients in overcoming their problems with automated task performance, because the dorsal visual

Table 8.2 Specific challenges for allied healthcare in atypical parkinsonism

	Parkinson's disease	Atypical parkinsonism
Evidence for allied health interventions	Greater amount of evidence, reflected by evidence-based guidelines	Small amount of evidence; depends on guidelines developed for PD
Expert opinion	Moderate, because of the high prevalence	Limited, because of low prevalence
Therapeutic options	Mainly extrapyramidal pathology: – permits bypass via intact cortical pathways, to compensate for hypokinetic symptoms – late development of life-threatening manifestations (falling, severe dysphagia) – cognitive impairment usually a late feature	More widespread disease pathology: – limited bypass via cortical pathways – early life-threatening manifestations (falling, severe dysphagia) – early and pronounced cognitive impairment
Disease progression	Usually slow; survival only mildly reduced	Usually rapid; survival markedly reduced

stream can bypass the defective basal ganglia and engage the primary motor cortex directly [13]. Furthermore, PD patients can be taught to execute complex movements by transforming the original task into a series of simple sub-movements that have to be executed consciously in a fixed sequential order [4]. Most treatment strategies in PD are based on these general principles. However, these strategies may be less effective for patients with AP when the alternative pathways also become damaged.

Second, the widespread disease pathology is responsible for a variety of motor symptoms that are not seen in patients with PD. These include the presence of spasticity, bulbar weakness, cerebellar ataxia, or apraxia. Treatment of these other motor symptoms requires a completely different approach compared to strategies to alleviate the hypokinetic features.

Another challenge is posed by the progressive nature of AP, which rapidly leads to increasing limitations. Hence, any improvements following intervention will likely deteriorate rather quickly with time, requiring periodic revisions to determine the need for renewed or adjusted treatment. However, good outcome measures are lacking for PD [14], let alone for patients with AP. On one hand, treatment should be stopped when there is no apparent benefit, thus avoiding an unnecessary burden placed on both the patient and the environment. On the other hand, particularly in patients with AP, problems may continue to worsen, even though treatment is actually effective; stopping the intervention will then further accelerate the disease process.

The rapid disease progression in AP also implies that allied health professionals have to address serious health risks at a much earlier stage compared to PD. Examples include repeated falling caused by severe postural instability, or the risk of unsafe nutrition and aspiration pneumonia caused by early, severe dysphagia.

Any treatment plan must consider the presence of cognitive impairment, which for most patients with AP is prominently present, even in an early stage of the disease (the main exception being patients with MSA, where cognitive decline is usually mild and generally develops late). Cognitive decline has implications for the ability of patients to understand the recommendations, and affects their capacity to apply the new movement strategies or techniques without the therapist being present. Other relevant factors to consider include depression and apathy, which affect the motivation of patients to participate in active treatment programs, or their willingness to apply newly learned strategies by themselves. This is why involvement of the immediate caregiver is often required, as was discussed previously.

Taken together, these considerations underscore the importance for the patient, their caregivers, and the allied health therapists of being aware of the limitations and challenges posed by the diagnosis of AP and of discussing realistic treatment goals.

Allied healthcare: more than just treatment

Allied health professionals can sometimes detect signs of AP before the medical specialist. For example, it may be an experienced speech–language therapist who is the first to notice subtle signs of speech ataxia in a patient who thus far was suspected of having PD. This may alert the medical team to the possible presence of AP, and perhaps warrant further ancillary studies. Similarly, physical therapists may be the first to detect signs of gait ataxia; for example, when tandem gait is tested under challenging conditions [15]. Signs of recklessness or an inability to acquire new motor skills may first come to light during therapeutic sessions with an occupational therapist. Occasionally they detect episodes of freezing when patients are observed while cooking dinner; for example, when a narrow turn has to be made in a small kitchen while carrying a tray with dishes. The importance of home visits has been mentioned where important new insights can be derived simply by observing how patients function in their own environment. As such, experienced allied health personnel can serve as a valuable diagnostic tool to recognize features of AP and support the medical specialist in establishing the proper diagnosis timeously.

Finally, allied health personnel witness patients under very different circumstances than do medical specialists, scoring and rating a very different part of the disease spectrum, namely disability and difficulties in participating in everyday activities. The medical specialist scores symptoms and signs, which is helpful in establishing a diagnosis, in scoring disease severity, and in evaluating the effects of drug therapy, for example. However, the severity of symptoms and signs often indicates little about what hinders the patient's experiences in daily life, because this depends also on the patient's preferences and coping strategies. It is surprising how well some clinically severely affected patients manage in a kitchen, for instance, or how poorly more mildly affected patients perform in daily life circumstances.

Outline for the remainder of this chapter

This chapter describes the key problems and treatment options of physical therapists, speech–language therapists, and occupational therapists when treating patients with AP. Most recommendations will be generically applicable to the mixed group of the various forms of AP. However, whenever possible, specific recommendations are provided for patients affected by PSP, MSA, corticobasal degeneration (CBD), dementia with Lewy bodies (DLB), or vascular parkinsonism (VP).

Physical therapy

Evidence-based practice guidelines are available for physical therapy in PD. A summary has been published [7] and the entire guideline is available (in English) via the website at *www.kngf.nl*. This guideline describes six specific core areas for physical therapy in PD (Table 8.3). In addition, the guideline describes four specific treatment recommendations that reach level 2 evidence. These core areas and therapeutic strategies are considered to be relevant also for the physical rehabilitation of patients with AP. As for patients with PD, it is recommended that most interventions take place at home because mobility problems are often related to the patient's home environment [12].

Gait

Similar to PD, gait in patients with AP can be disturbed in two ways: abnormalities that are present continuously, and features that are seen only episodically [16]. For most patients with AP, the continuous gait disturbance is dominated by hypokinetic-rigid features that can resemble the gait of PD patients: a reduced stride length that is compensated by an increased step frequency; a diminished step height, which increases the risk of stumbling; a reduced walking speed, partially reflecting gait bradykinesia but perhaps also reflecting a purposeful slowing to render gait safer; and decreased trunk rotation, for example, while turning around (*en bloc* turning). However, there are also differences: arm swing, which is asymmetrically reduced in PD, more symmetrically absent in AP, but can be relatively preserved in VP. An asymmetrical arm swing is also seen in CBD where it is usually accompanied by early and relatively fixed hand or foot dystonia. Typical for patients with AP is their wide-based gait, which would be unusual for patients with PD. This wide-based gait in AP may reflect underlying cerebellar or other extra-nigral pathology, or an attempt to compensate for a perceived balance deficit. Tandem gait (tested by asking patients to make 10 consecutive tandem steps) remains intact until late-stage PD, but typically becomes abnormal in early stages of AP [15].

The episodic gait disturbance is only present periodically, typically under specific circumstances such as turning around, while crossing a narrow passage, or during dual tasking [16,17]. The best characterized episodic gait disturbance is called freezing of gait (FOG), defined as an inability to generate effective forward stepping movements that are accompanied by a characteristic feeling of the feet becoming glued to the floor [18,19]. Festination is defined as rapidly taking increasingly small steps (hastening) to avoid a fall, but without

Table 8.3 Indications for referring patients with atypical parkinsonism to a physical therapist [7]

Presence of
• (risk of) physical inactivity
• fear of moving or falling
• limitations in transfers
• limitations in walking, including freezing of gait
• postural instability and falls
• problems with body posture, reaching, and grasping
• (risk of) physical incapacity and reduced joint mobility

the feeling of gluing. Often FOG is an early symptom that can be present in all forms of AP except neuroleptic-induced parkinsonism.

When hypokinesia is the most prominent feature, gait in patients with AP can be improved by applying visual, auditory, tactile, or mental cues, or by using cognitive movement strategies [12,13,20–22]. Although the evidence was obtained only for PD, it is suggested that these strategies can also partially benefit gait in patients with AP, as long as the (cortical) bypasses for the basal ganglia remain intact. The effects are usually more modest and short-lasting compared to PD, and a sizeable subgroup does not benefit at all. Depending on the extent of the additional neurological impairments, gait can be improved by training trunk mobility and by leg muscle strengthening [7,23]. Further instructions can be given concerning arm swing, base of support, heel contact, and step size [21,24]. Finally, it is important to train the patient in the use of assistive devices, such as walking frames or wheeled rollators.

Transfers

Many patients with parkinsonism perceive problems in performing transfers such as rising from a chair or rolling over in bed [25]. Cognitive movement strategies can be used to improve such transfers, by splitting complex (automatic) movements into a series of relatively simple movement elements that are consciously executed in a defined sequence [12,26]. Again, all available evidence stems from PD, but these strategies can certainly benefit patients with AP. Dual tasking during complex (automatic) transfers should be avoided, and transfers can be guided using external cues to facilitate movement initiation [22,27]. Obviously these adaptations should also be practiced in the patient's own environment and with the assistance of instructed caregivers.

Balance and falls

Progressive postural instability is a common problem for patients with AP, and recurrent falls can be an early sign [6]. The prevalence of recurrent falls is high, up to 100% in PSP patients, and falls occurring shortly after disease onset represent a clear red flag as against a diagnosis of PD (and as such alert the physical therapist) [3]. Latency to onset of recurrents falls is short for PSP (6 months), intermediate for MSA, DLB, and CBD (24–48 months), and long for PD (118 months) [3].

Most falls are intrinsic, caused by patient-related factors such as freezing during turning or poor balance reactions when being perturbed. However, extrinsic (or environmental) factors such as narrow doorways or slippery floors may also play a role, so it may be useful to pay a home visit and remove obvious domestic hazards. Exercises to improve balance and to prevent falls are effective in PD [28], and may also benefit patients with AP. In addition, advice and information can be given concerning footwear and how to deal with orthostatic hypotension [17,29]. Preventing falls in the elderly is most effective when a multidisciplinary team approach is used, but whether this is also true for PD or AP remains to be investigated [30].

Body posture

Posture is typically stooped in most AP syndromes, except in PSP where patients are more likely to demonstrate an erect posture with retrocollis. MSA patients often combine a stooped posture with antecollis or laterocollis, as well as lateral bending of the trunk (Pisa syndrome). Additionally, reduced trunk flexibility is often present. Exercise programs that focus on the coordination of muscle activity while maintaining posture and movement can facilitate performance of skills and activities such as grasping, rolling over in bed, or preserving balance [31,32]. Additionally, the changes in posture can be corrected by applying verbal or visual feedback; for example, using a mirror [24].

Reaching and grasping

Several techniques can be used to improve the ability to reach, grasp, and manipulate objects. This includes cueing strategies to initiate and continue activities, cognitive movement strategies, and avoidance of dual tasking [33]. However, other compensations should be applied when additional neurological abnormalities are present, such as spasticity or ideomotor apraxia, especially to avoid risky situations.

Physical inactivity

PD patients tend to be inactive, and this is probably also true of patients with AP. Physical inactivity may cause a host of secondary complications such as decreased aerobic capacity, muscle weakness, joint problems, and osteoporosis [16]. Therefore, patients should be informed about the health benefits of exercise and be encouraged to participate in sports, but obviously in a safe context [34]. Given the early loss of independent ambulation and faster disease progression, careful guidance and professional advice is needed for patients with AP.

Speech–language therapy

A guideline of speech–language therapy in PD has recently been published [9,35] with recommendations for clinical practice, but currently this is only available in the Dutch language. A translation into English is underway.

Speech–language therapy for patients with AP focuses on three domains: dysarthria (speech and voice impairment), dysphagia (swallowing disorders), and drooling (involuntary saliva loss) (Table 8.4). Unlike in PD, dysarthria and dysphagia typically are early symptoms in AP. For example, the prevalence of Hypophonia in PD is estimated at about 70% [36], while in AP virtually all patients are affected [37,38]. The prevalence of dysphagia in PD is approximately 50% [39], but much higher rates are reported for PSP and MSA [38]. In addition, unintelligible speech and severe dysphagia are two of the clinical milestones when studying the disease progression of PSP and MSA [40,41]. The prevalence of drooling in PD has been studied only superficially and estimated at about 56% [42], but is hardly documented in AP. One study in patients with PSP reported a prevalence of 63% [43]; thus, drooling appears at least as common in PSP.

Table 8.4 Indications for referring patients with atypical parkinsonism to a speech–language therapist [9]

- presence of limitations in speech and verbal communication
- presence of limitations in swallowing capacity (possibly causing drooling) or problems with eating and drinking owing to a swallowing disorder (possibly causing aspiration pneumonia or unwanted weight loss)
- need for advice and training in use of communication aids

Table 8.5 Features of hypokinetic, spastic, flaccid, and ataxic dysarthria [44,46]

Speech dimensions	Hypokinetic	Spastic	Flaccid	Ataxic
Breathing	shallow, reduced exhalation control	shallow, slow, antagonist muscular contractions	shallow, slow, reduced pressure generation	shallow, irregular and sudden-forced patterns
Voice quality	low volume, hoarse or breathy quality, high pitched, difficulty initiating phonation	strained-strangled, harsh, low pitched	hoarse, breathy, reduced pitch and loudness, audible inspirations	hoarse, breathy, variable
Articulation	small articulatory movements, mumbling	slow-laboured, imprecise	slow-laboured, imprecise	imprecise, slow, irregular
Resonance	normal	normal to hyponasal	hypernasal, nasal emissions	variable
Prosody	monopitch and monoloudness	monoloudness	reduced pitch and loudness variations	explosive syllable stress, loudness and pitch outbursts, abnormal prolongations of phonemes
Speech rate	normal to high	low, short phrases	low, short phrases	variable

Dysarthria

Characteristic for speech impairment in AP is a mixed dysarthria, meaning that hypokinetic dysarthria is combined with spastic, flaccid, or ataxic features [44–46]. PSP patients usually demonstrate a hypokinetic-spastic dysarthria, but ataxic dysarthria can be present as well [47]. In MSA patients, the speech impairment can be a combination of hypokinetic, ataxic, flaccid, and spastic dysarthria, with hypokinetic dysarthria as the dominant type in MSA-P, and ataxic dysarthria as the most striking feature in MSA-C [48]. Patients with CBD usually have a hypokinetic-spastic dysarthria, but apraxia of speech can also be present [49,50]. Dysarthric features in patients with DLB or VP are less well described. Recognizing the various components of speech impairment is notoriously difficult, and requires a great deal of expertise. Previously, it was alluded that experienced speech–language therapists are able to support the neurological diagnosis with careful motor speech examination and identification of specific dysarthric features (Table 8.5).

Dysarthria can have a great impact on the quality of life [51]. It is associated with a reduced intelligibility, interfering with the ability to communicate with others. This impaired communication is further aggravated by the loss of facial expression (hypomimia or mask face), another manifestation of hypokinesia.

There is good evidence (level 2) that specific treatment of hypokinetic dysarthria in PD patients is successful. The Lee Silverman Voice Treatment (LSVT) is an effective therapy to overcome the hypokinetic voice production and small articulation movements by learning to speak louder [52]. This is possible mainly through intensive training (four times a week, for four weeks), and improved quality of speech can be maintained for more than a year [53]. A comparable approach, the Pitch Limiting Voice Treatment (PLVT) also improves loudness and voice quality, but at the same time limits the increase in vocal pitch that usually occurs when loudness is increased [54]. Although both techniques have been evaluated only in patients with mild to moderate PD, these interventions can also be useful in AP patients when the dysarthria is dominated by hypokinetic features. Clinicians need to make sure that patients indeed respond well to cueing to improve speech intelligibility, and also have the physical and cognitive abilities to cooperate in an intensive treatment. This requires good cooperation with other professionals involved in the care of each individual patient, to avoid excessive strain on the patient and the environment. Advanced patients are likely to remain dependent on caregivers for providing the cues, and the results are generally modest. High-intensity techniques are contraindicated when spastic or ataxic features are more prominent, because putting in more energy will typically worsen breathing, voice quality, and normalcy of speech.

Spastic, flaccid, and ataxic speech characteristics call for different interventions. Although, in general, the management of motor speech disorders lags behind description and understanding [44], many interventions have been developed [46]. Indirect techniques include strengthening exercises, improving the altered posture and positioning, or relaxation exercises. Behavioral treatment can focus either on modification of respiration, phonation, and articulation, or on improvement of efficiency and naturalness. When the need to communicate is particularly frustrated by unintelligible speech, augmentative and alternative communication (AAC) might be an option. The development of AAC thrives on the expansion of electronic and computer-based technology, including synthesized speech. However, some form of volitional motor behavior and cognitive ability is always needed to handle any communication aid and produce comprehensible output. That makes MSA patients the most likely candidates for successful application. A specific tool that is sometimes requested by soft-speaking parkinsonism patients is a (portable) amplification system, to enhance their speech volume. This device is only helpful if speech is still sufficiently intelligible.

Dysphagia

In patients with PD, dysphagia improves only partly with the use of levodopa [55] or deep brain stimulation [56]. This suggests that even in PD, dysphagia results at least in part from changes in non-dopaminergic mechanisms, like the medullary central pattern generator for swallowing [55,57]. This is certainly true for patients with AP; severe swallowing disorders can be observed even in the early stages of PSP or MSA, for example [43,58]. In general, oropharyngeal dysphagia increases the risk of aspiration of oral secretions or food, which can result in pneumonia. Combined with a reduced cough reflex sensitivity and a diminished cough intensity (which deteriorate with advancing parkinsonism), silent aspiration and aspiration pneumonia are serious risks [59]. In the end-of-life stage, (aspiration) pneumonia is one of the main causes of death [60,61]. Inability to participate in joint meals with family or friends as a result of severe dysphagia also has great social implications [62].

Mild dysphagia in patients with parkinsonism can usually be compensated successfully with techniques that are regularly applied by speech therapists [9,63]. The main goals are prevention of aspiration and comfortable and sufficient oral intake. Aspiration of liquids resulting from a delayed pharyngeal swallow can be avoided by applying a chin-down posture during swallowing to protect the airway entrance from premature liquid flow [64]. A typical solution in patients with parkinsonism is avoiding dual tasking: drinking or eating while having a conversation. Swallowing smaller-sized amounts is another uselful compensation to prevent aspiration, but might be contraindicated for patients who need a substantial food or liquid bolus to start swallowing because of decreased oral sensitivity (for example, in PSP or VP), especially when akinesia makes it difficult to induce a swallow. Difficulties with swallowing solid food can be overcome by swallowing with more effort (instructing patients to swallow hard), similar to speaking more loudly, when hypokinesia is the main cause. Treatment becomes particularly challenging when chewing is also problematic, when patients have difficulty swallowing their medication, or when mealtimes become extremely long. In such patients, it is useful for the speech therapist to observe the patients at home and to find specific instructions and cues that can be applied in their own environments.

More severe dysphagia complaints call for modification of food consistencies, but care should be taken to retain taste, appearance, nutritional standards, and individual and cultural preferences [63]. Help of an experienced dietician is recommended in these cases, and also when nutritional supplements are considered. Enteral feeding via percutaneous endoscopic gastrostomy (PEG) is seldom needed in PD patients, but more commonly used in patients with PSP or MSA [40,60] when safe swallowing is severely compromised and oral intake has become insufficient [65]. There are no accepted indications to start enteral feeding in patients with AP, but this approach should be considered when malnutrition, weight loss, and aspiration risk can no longer be resisted by the behavioral interventions described previously, or when oral feeding takes more than reasonable effort and time from the patients and their caregivers.

Drooling

The pathophysiology of drooling remains insufficiently understood. Hypersalivation (increased saliva production) was long held responsible, but recent work suggests that this is an unlikely cause; several studies have now confirmed that salivary flow in PD patients is not increased and in fact even lower compared to controls [66]. Drooling is more likely to be caused by infrequent swallowing and involuntary mouth opening as part of the facial masking. In addition, antecollis – as seen in some MSA patients – and a stooped posture will contribute as well, because gravity promotes dripping of saliva. Drooling is often hard to observe during a therapeutic session because PD patients tend to drool mainly when they are unobserved or distracted by a non-verbal activity.

Behavioral treatments are limited. Mild drooling can be diminished by practicing the habit of swallowing saliva before starting to speak or before standing up, but the success depends on the patient's cognitive abilities. For more severe cases, pharmacological treatment is recommended. Botulinum toxin injections into the salivary glands are applied most often [67]. Alternative approaches include the use of systemic or topical anticholinergic drugs or, as a last-resort treatment, radiotherapy applied over the salivary glands.

Occupational therapy

A guideline of occupational therapy in PD has been published recently [8,68] with recommendations for clinical practice, but currently this is only available in the Dutch language. A translation into English is underway.

The primary role of occupational therapy is enabling occupation, best defined as everything people are engaged in, including looking after themselves (self-care), enjoying life (leisure), and contributing to the social or economic fabric of their communities (productivity). In order to optimize occupational performance and participation (and the patient's satisfaction with occupational performance), interventions applied by occupational therapists can focus on: changing aspects of the person (either the patient or the caregiver), the actual activities, and the environment where the activities are performed. Although occupational therapy and physical therapy are closely related, there is a clear difference between the therapies with respect to their core areas. Physical therapy is directed to improving basic skills such as gait or transfers, thereby aiming to improve daily functioning. In contrast, occupational therapy is focused more on being able to use these skills, allowing subjects to perform complex activities such as gardening, shopping, or working at a computer.

For patients with AP, occupational therapy aims to reduce limitations in participation or daily activities that can be ascribed to the motor and non-motor disabilities of their parkinsonism. Independence in performing daily activities is the goal in early-stage disease. However, for patients with severe limitations in performing daily activities, the focus shifts toward enabling an adapted involvement in activities (occupational engagement).

Occupational therapists use comprehensive clinical assessments to uncover the needs of the patients and their caregivers, and to analyze which factors limit or support occupational performance and participation. Table 8.6 shows several indications for referral to an occupational therapist [8,10].

There is some evidence that occupational therapy can improve functional abilities in mildly to moderately affected MSA patients [69]. Other than that, currently there is no good evidence to support the use of occupational therapy in either PD or AP. Most recommendations for the treatment of patients with parkinsonism therefore are based on insights and evidence derived from other chronic disorders with functional problems that resemble those seen in parkinsonism. Again, occupational therapy strategies are preferably applied in the patient's own home environment [12].

Improving limitations in participation and activities

Occupational therapy interventions in PD include teaching patients alternative and compensatory strategies to improve their task performance. The recently developed evidence-based

Table 8.6 Indications for referring patients with atypical parkinsonism to an occupational therapist [8]

The patient experiences limitations in activities and participation in the following domains
• self-care, family care and functional mobility
• productivity (paid and unpaid work)
• leisure activities
The caregiver expresses problems in the care for the patient in daily activities
The physician questions the safety and independence of the patient while performing daily activities

guideline for occupational therapy in PD recommends 10 strategies, most of which may also be applicable to patients with AP [10]. Three compensatory motor strategies are specific for parkinsonism and are shared with the other allied health professionals: avoiding multitasking during daily activities [33], using cues to initiate and maintain movements during activities [13,70], and using cognitive movement strategies to break down complex performance sequences of activities into simple movement elements [4,12,26]. The presence of spasticity, ataxia, or severe cognitive decline may limit the effect of these strategies, which were designed specifically to compensate for hypokinesia and bradykinesia. Ideomotor apraxia may also be present, especially in patients with PSP, CBD, or VP. This apraxia can manifest itself during complex activities, and it necessitates cognitive compensatory strategies that are currently used for apraxia in stroke [71,72]. Simplifying activities, advice about alternative equipment, or making changes to the physical environment are frequently used interventions.

Another treatment strategy usually applied by occupational therapists is optimizing the planning of daily and weekly routines. This planning carefully considers the patient's energy levels, medication effects (for example, planning shopping during the ON phase), the preferred activities, and the speed of task performance [73,74]. The scheme also provides structure to prompt timely initiation of activities. This may include explicitly reducing stress and minimizing time pressure while performing activities.

An essential element in the approach by occupational therapists is to address the needs of caregivers on issues related to activities and participation, especially for patients with AP who largely depend on the help and support of informal caregivers. This is done by providing caregivers with information, advice, and training. These interventions can improve their way of coping with complex situations and their competence in supporting the patient [75–77]. Finally, for both patients and caregivers, encouraging self-management skills throughout the treatment process is a basis for learning to deal with problems [78,79].

Other non-pharmacological treatments

There is a variety of additional non-pharmacological strategies that help to support patients with AP. These will be addressed only briefly here. Unwanted weight loss or malnutrition is common in AP. There are several possible causes, including dysphagia, depression, and loss of appetite (owing to hyposmia or because of nausea as a side-effect of medication) [80,81]. A dietician can help to optimize the nutritional status of patients. Another important role is to coach patients in avoiding high-protein meals together with the intake of medication because proteins can interfere with the gastrointestinal absorption of levodopa, for instance [82]. Promoting an adequate fluid intake may help to reduce constipation, and may also alleviate orthostatic hypotension. Urinary incontinence may worsen, and nocturia particularly is cumbersome for patients. Such patients should be advised to drink mostly during the day and to avoid coffee and alcoholic beverages in the evening.

Social workers are increasingly engaged as part of the multidisciplinary team. Target areas where social workers can provide support include disease acceptance and coping, relational aspects, and support of the financial situation; for example, in patients with pathological gambling.

Sexual dysfunction is common in patients with AP, affecting both women and men [83]. In addition to adjusting the medical treatment regime (implemented by the neurologist), sexologists have an important counseling function for both patients and their partners; for example, by discussing the use of supportive aids to improve sexual functioning.

Multidisciplinary approach

In many countries, allied healthcare is prescribed commonly for patients with PD and AP. Moreover, integrated multidisciplinary care programs are increasingly implemented in specialized Parkinson centers, hoping that provision of integrated non-pharmacological management helps to support patients and their caregivers optimally [4]. Using a multi-disciplinary team approach requires that the participating health professionals are aware of the treatment options that potentially can be delivered by the other team members. Allied health specialists must also be willing to exchange information with each other and with the medical specialists [5].

Toward better implementation in clinical practice

Unfortunately, current delivery of allied healthcare services remains inadequate in several respects. Many patients who require allied care are not being referred, whereas other patients do receive care on questionable grounds or are being treated for unnecessarily long periods of time. For example, a recent survey in the Netherlands among PD patients showed that referral rates were only 9% for occupational therapy and 14% for speech–language therapy [84]. This unsatisfactory situation can be explained partly by: the lack of strong scientific evidence for most allied healthcare interventions; the limited knowledge and sometimes scepticism among medical doctors (neurologists, geriatricians, or general practitioners) about the added value of allied healthcare for patients with PD or AP; the absence of specific expertise among most allied health therapists partly because of the small volume of patients with parkinsonism treated annually by each individual therapist [25,84]; and the generally poor communication between healthcare providers involved in the care of patients with PD or AP (for example, between physical therapists and referring neurologists). These factors might well keep physicians from referring their patients, and also explain why treatment is suboptimal for those patients who are being referred.

One option to tackle these problems is the development of community-based networks of dedicated health professionals specialized in parkinsonism. Such regional networks have been introduced recently in the Netherlands under the name ParkinsonNet [11,85]. The central idea is that – within a given region – patients should be treated preferentially by a small group of selected professionals with a high degree of expertise in both PD and AP. This expertise is gained initially during an intensive training course, and is maintained at a high level because patients are being referred specifically to these ParkinsonNet therapists. Consequently, their treatment volume increases considerably, allowing therapists to apply and extend their expertise in clinical practice continually. Furthermore, the participating allied health professionals receive continuous education, supported by a web-based training and communication facility. Finally, an electronic patient record (EPR) is used, which supports clinical decision making based on the clinical guidelines as described previously. The ParkinsonNet concept assumes an active role for patients and their families (patient empowerment); for example, by using a simple screening tool for self-assessment and self-referral, and by clarifying for patients where the ParkinsonNet therapists can be found in their region. Patients also have access to their own EPR. Further important elements of this ParkinsonNet concept include improved communication among all health professionals and structuring of the referral process (by promoting dedicated referrals to ParkinsonNet therapists). The merits of this ParkinsonNet concept have been evaluated recently in a large cluster-randomized study (the ParkinsonNet trial) involving around 700 patients with PD (patients with AP were excluded) [85]. The first results suggest that the treatment volume per therapist increases from around 4 to more than 12 patients per year, that the quality of care increases, while the costs for society decrease. A major challenge that now lies ahead is to demonstrate that such an optimized delivery of allied health interventions will help to maintain independence and improve the quality of life of patients with AP.

Acknowledgments

We thank Bert de Swart, speech pathologist, Ingrid Sturkenboom, occupational therapist, and Maarten Nijkrake, physical therapist for sharing their expertise with us. Professor Bastiaan R Bloem was supported by a ZonMw VIDI research grant (number 016.076.352).

References

1. Bloem BR, Bhatia KP. Gait and balance in basal ganglia disorders. In: Bronstein AM, Brandt T, Nutt JG, Woollacott MH, eds. *Clinical Disorders of Balance, Posture and Gait*. London: Arnold, 2004; 173–206.

2. Litvan I, Grimes DA, Lang AE, et al. Clinical features differentiating patients with postmortem confirmed progressive supranuclear palsy and corticobasal degeneration. *J Neurol* 1999; **246**(Suppl 2): II1–5.

3. Wenning GK, Ebersbach G, Verny M, et al. Progression of falls in postmortem-confirmed parkinsonian disorders. *Mov Disord* 1999; **14**(6): 947–50.

4. Morris MS, Iansek RN. *Parkinson's disease: a team approach*. Melbourne, Australia: Buscombe Vicprint, 1997.

5. Deane KH, Ellis-Hill C, Jones D, et al. Systematic review of paramedical therapies for Parkinson's disease. *Mov Disord* 2002; **17**(5): 984–91.

6. Houghton DJ, Litvan I. Unraveling progressive supranuclear palsy: from the bedside back to the bench. *Parkinsonism Relat Disord* 2007; **13**(Suppl 3): S341–346.

7. Keus SH, Bloem BR, Hendriks EJ, et al. Evidence-based analysis of physical therapy in Parkinson's disease with recommendations for practice and research. *Mov Disord* 2007; **22**(4): 451–60.

8. Sturkenboom IHWM, Kalf JG, Bloem BR, et al. Guidelines for occupational therapy in Parkinson's disease. *Mov Disord* 2008; **23**: S329.

9. Kalf JG, de Swart BJM, Bloem BR, et al. Guidelines for speech-language therapy in Parkinson's disease. *Mov Disord* 2008; **23**: S328.

10. Kalf H, Sturkenboom I, Thijssen M, et al. Pursuing best practice in multidisciplinary care. *EPNN J* 2008; 14: 12–15.

11. Nijkrake MJ, Keus SHJ, Kalf JG, et al. Allied health care interventions and complementary therapies in Parkinson's disease. *Parkinsonism Rel Disord* 2007; **13**(Suppl 3): S488–94.

12. Nieuwboer A, De WW, Dom R, et al. The effect of a home physiotherapy program for persons with Parkinson's disease. *J Rehabil Med* 2001; **33**(6): 266–72.

13. Nieuwboer A, Kwakkel G, Rochester L, et al. Cueing training in the home improves gait-related mobility in Parkinson's disease: the RESCUE trial. *J Neurol Neurosurg Psychiatry* 2007; **78**(2): 134–40.

14. Keus SH, Munneke M, Nijkrake MJ, et al. Physical therapy in Parkinson's disease: evolution and future challenges. *Mov Disord* 2009; **24**(1): 1–14.

15. Abdo WF, Borm GF, Munneke M, et al. Ten steps to identify atypical parkinsonism. *J Neurol Neurosurg Psychiatry* 2006; **77**(12): 1367–9.

16. Snijders AH, van de Warrenburg BP, Giladi N, et al. Neurological gait disorders in elderly people: clinical approach and classification. *Lancet Neurol* 2007; **6**(1): 63–74.

17. Morris ME. Locomotor training in people with Parkinson disease. *Phys Ther* 2006; **86**(10): 1426–35.

18. Nieuwboer A, Giladi N. The challenge of evaluating freezing of gait in patients with

Parkinson's disease. *Br J Neurosurg* 2008; **22**(Suppl 1): S16–18.

19. Snijders AH, Nijkrake MJ, Bakker M, et al. Clinimetrics of freezing of gait. *Mov Disord* 2008; **23**(Suppl 2): S468–74.

20. Thaut MH, McIntosh GC, Rice RR, et al. Rhythmic auditory stimulation in gait training for Parkinson's disease patients. *Mov Disord* 1996; **11**(2): 193–200.

21. Behrman AL, Teitelbaum P, Cauraugh JH. Verbal instructional sets to normalise the temporal and spatial gait variables in Parkinson's disease. *J Neurol Neurosurg Psychiatry* 1998; **65**(4): 580–2.

22. Muller V, Mohr B, Rosin R, et al. Short-term effects of behavioral treatment on movement initiation and postural control in Parkinson's disease: a controlled clinical study. *Mov Disord* 1997; **12**(3): 306–14.

23. Scandalis TA, Bosak A, Berliner JC, et al. Resistance training and gait function in patients with Parkinson's disease. *Am J Phys Med Rehabil* 2001; **80**(1): 38–43.

24. Formisano R, Pratesi L, Modarelli FT, et al . Rehabilitation and Parkinson's disease. *Scand J Rehabil Med* 1992; **24**(3): 157–60.

25. Keus SH, Bloem BR, Verbaan D, et al. Physiotherapy in Parkinson's disease: utilisation and patient satisfaction. *J Neurol* 2004; **251**(6): 680–7.

26. Kamsma YPT, Brouwer WH, Lakke JPW. Training of compensational strategies for impaired gross motor skills in Parkinson's disease. *Physiother Theory Pract* 1995; **11**: 209–29.

27. Mak MK, Hui-Chan CW. Audiovisual cues can enhance sit-to-stand in patients with Parkinson's disease. *Mov Disord* 2004; **19**(9): 1012–19.

28. Toole T, Hirsch MA, Forkink A, et al. The effects of a balance and strength training program on equilibrium in Parkinsonism: A preliminary study. *NeuroRehabilitation* 2000; **14**(3): 165–74.

29. Constantinescu R, Leonard C, Deeley C, et al. Assistive devices for gait in Parkinson's disease. *Parkinsonism Relat Disord* 2007; **13**(3): 133–8.

30. Gillespie LD, Gillespie WJ, Robertson MC, et al. Interventions for preventing falls in elderly people. *Cochrane Database Syst Rev* 2003; **4**: CD000340.

31. Stallibrass C, Sissons P, Chalmers C. Randomized controlled trial of the Alexander technique for idiopathic Parkinson's disease. *Clin Rehabil* 2002; **16**(7): 695–708.

32. Schenkman M, Cutson TM, Kuchibhatla M, et al. Exercise to improve spinal flexibility and function for people with Parkinson's disease: a randomized, controlled trial. *J Am Geriatr Soc* 1998; **46**(10): 1207–16.

33. Morris ME. Movement disorders in people with Parkinson disease: a model for physical therapy. *Phys Ther* 2000; **80**(6): 578–97.

34. Crizzle AM, Newhouse IJ. Is physical exercise beneficial for persons with Parkinson's disease? *Clin J Sport Med* 2006; **16**(5): 422–5.

35. Kalf JG, de Swart BJM, Bonnier MWJ, et al. Logopedie bij de ziekte van Parkinson. Een richtlijn van de Nederlandse Vereniging voor Logopedie en Foniatrie. *Woerden: NVLF/Uitgeverij LEMMA*, 2008.

36. Ho AK, Iansek R, Marigliani C, et al. Speech impairment in a large sample of patients with Parkinson's disease. *Behav Neurol* 1998; **11**(3): 131–7.

37. Litvan I, Mangone CA, McKee A, et al. Natural history of progressive supranuclear palsy (Steele–Richardson–Olszewski syndrome) and clinical predictors of survival: a clinicopathological study. *J Neurol Neurosurg Psychiatry* 1996; **60**(6): 615–20.

38. Muller J, Wenning GK, Verny M, et al. Progression of dysarthria and dysphagia in postmortem-confirmed parkinsonian disorders. *Arch Neurol* 2001; **58**(2): 259–64.

39. Johnston BT, Li Q, Castell JA, et al. Swallowing and esophageal function in Parkinson's disease. *Am J Gastroenterol* 1995; **90**(10): 1741–6.

40. Goetz CG, Leurgans S, Lang AE, et al. Progression of gait, speech and swallowing deficits in progressive supranuclear palsy. *Neurology* 2003; **60**(6): 917–22.

41. O'Sullivan SS, Massey LA, Williams DR, et al. Clinical outcomes of progressive supranuclear palsy and multiple system atrophy. *Brain* 2008; **131**(5): 1362–72.

42. Kalf JG, de Swart BJM, Borm GF, et al. Prevalence and definition of drooling in

Parkinson's disease: a systematic review. *J Neurol* 2009; **256**(9): 1391–6.

43. Litvan I, Sastry N, Sonies BC. Characterizing swallowing abnormalities in progressive supranuclear palsy. *Neurology* 1997; **48**(6): 1654–62.

44. Duffy JR. *Motor Speech Disorders. Substrates, differential diagnosis and management.* St Louis: Elsevier Mosby, 2005.

45. Sachin S, Shukla G, Goyal V, et al. Clinical speech impairment in Parkinson's disease, progressive supranuclear palsy, and multiple system atrophy. *Neurol India* 2008; **56**(2): 122–6.

46. Dworkin JP. *Motor Speech Disorders. A Treatment Guide.* St. Louis: Mosby – Year Book, Inc., 1991.

47. Kluin K, Gilman S, Foster N, et al. Neuropathological correlates of dysarthria in progressive supranuclear palsy. *Arch Neurol* 2001; **58**(2): 265–9.

48. Kluin KJ, Gilman S, Lohman M, et al. Characteristics of the dysarthria of multiple system atrophy. *Arch Neurol* 1996; **53**(6): 545–8.

49. Ozsancak C, Auzou P, Hannequin D. Dysarthria and orofacial apraxia in corticobasal degeneration. *Mov Disord* 2000; **15**(5): 905–10.

50. Ozsancak C, Auzou P, Dujardin K, et al. Orofacial apraxia in corticobasal degeneration, progressive supranuclear palsy, multiple system atrophy and Parkinson's disease. *J Neurol* 2004; **251**(11): 1317–23.

51. Miller N, Noble E, Jones D, et al. Life with communication changes in Parkinson's disease. *Age Ageing* 2006; **35**(3): 235–9.

52. Ramig LO, Countryman S, Thompson LL, et al. Comparison of two forms of intensive speech treatment for Parkinson disease. *J Speech Hear Res* 1995; **38**(6): 1232–51.

53. Ramig LO, Countryman S, O'Brien C, et al. Intensive speech treatment for patients with Parkinson's disease: short- and long-term comparison of two techniques. *Neurology* 1996; **47**(6): 1496–504.

54. Swart de BJ, Willemse SC, Maassen BA, et al. Improvement of voicing in patients with Parkinson's disease by speech therapy. *Neurology* 2003; **60**(3): 498–500.

55. Hunter PC, Crameri J, Austin S, et al. Response of parkinsonian swallowing dysfunction to dopaminergic stimulation. *J Neurol Neurosurg Psychiatry* 1997; **63**(5): 579–83.

56. Ciucci MR, Barkmeier-Kraemer JM, Sherman SJ. Subthalamic nucleus deep brain stimulation improves deglutition in Parkinson's disease. *Mov Disord* 2008; **23**(5): 676–83.

57. Alfonsi E, Versino M, Merlo IM, et al. Electrophysiologic patterns of oral-pharyngeal swallowing in parkinsonian syndromes. *Neurology* 2007; **68**(8): 583–9.

58. Nath U, Ben-Shlomo Y, Thomson RG, et al. Clinical features and natural history of progressive supranuclear palsy: a clinical cohort study. *Neurology* 2003; **60**(6): 892–3.

59. Ebihara S, Saito H, Kanda A, et al. Impaired efficacy of cough in patients with Parkinson disease. *Chest* 2003; **124**(3): 1009–15.

60. Papapetropoulos S, Singer C, McCorquodale D, et al. Cause, seasonality of death and co-morbidities in progressive supranuclear palsy (PSP). *Parkinsonism Relat Disord* 2005; **11**(7): 459–63.

61. Wenning GK, Tison F, Ben SY, et al. Multiple system atrophy: a review of 203 pathologically proven cases. *Mov Disord* 1997; **12**(2): 133–47.

62. Miller N, Noble E, Jones D, et al. Hard to swallow: dysphagia in Parkinson's disease. *Age Ageing* 2006; **35**(6): 614–18.

63. Huckabee ML, Pelletier CA. *Management of Adult Neurogenic Dysphagia.* New York: Thomson Delmar Learning, 2003.

64. Welch MV, Logemann JA, Rademaker AW, et al. Changes in pharyngeal dimensions effected by chin tuck. *Arch Phys Med Rehabil* 1993; **74**(2): 178–81.

65. Perlman AL, Schulze-Delrieu KS. *Deglutition and its Disorders.* San Diego: Singular Publishing Group, 1997.

66. Tumilasci OR, Cersosimo MG, Belforte JE, et al. Quantitative study of salivary secretion in Parkinson's disease. *Mov Disord* 2006; **21**(5): 660–7.

67. Chou KL, Evatt M, Hinson V, et al. Sialorrhea in Parkinson's disease: a review. *Mov Disord* 2007; **22**(16): 2306–13.

68. Sturkenboom IHWM, Thijssen MCE, Gons-van Elsacker JJ, et al. Ergotherapie bij de ziekte van Parkinson. Een richtlijn van Ergotherapie Nederland.

Utrecht: Ergotherapie Nederland/Uitgeverij LEMMA, 2008.

69. Jain S, Dawson J, Quinn NP, et al. Occupational therapy in multiple system atrophy: a pilot randomized controlled trial. *Mov Disord* 2004; **19**(11): 1360–4.

70. Oliveira RM, Gurd JM, Nixon P, et al. Micrographia in Parkinson's disease: the effect of providing external cues. *J Neurol Neurosurg Psychiatry* 1997; **63**(4): 429–33.

71. Pharr V, Uttl B, Stark M, et al. Comparison of apraxia in corticobasal degeneration and progressive supranuclear palsy. *Neurology* 2001; **56**(7): 957–63.

72. van Heugten CM, Dekker J, Deelman BG, et al. Outcome of strategy training in stroke patients with apraxia: a phase II study. *Clin Rehabil* 1998; **12**(4): 294–303.

73. Landes AM, Sperry SD, Strauss ME, et al. Apathy in Alzheimer's disease. *J Am Geriatr Soc* 2001; **49**(12): 1700–7.

74. Matuska K, Mathiowetz V, Finlayson M. Use and perceived effectiveness of energy conservation strategies for managing multiple sclerosis fatigue. *Am J Occup Ther* 2007; **61**(1): 62–9.

75. Gitlin LN, Winter L, Corcoran M, et al. Effects of the home environmental skill-building program on the caregiver-care recipient dyad: 6-month outcomes from the Philadelphia REACH Initiative. *Gerontologist* 2003; **43**(4): 532–46.

76. Gitlin LN, Hauck WW, Dennis MP, et al. Maintenance of effects of the home environmental skill-building program for family caregivers and individuals with Alzheimer's disease and related disorders. *J Gerontol A Biol Sci Med Sci* 2005; **60**(3): 368–74.

77. Graff MJ, Vernooij-Dassen MJ, Thijssen M, et al. Community based occupational therapy for patients with dementia and their care givers: randomised controlled trial. *BMJ* 2006; **333**(7580): 1196.

78. Sutter D, Curdt T, Neufeld P. Promoting community participation among persons with Parkinson's and their caregivers: occupational therapy practitioners can facilitate persons with Parkinson's disease finding ways to continue to participate in valued occupation. *OT Practice* 2006; **11**: 19–22.

79. Simons G, Thompson SB, Smith Pasqualini MC. An innovative education programme for people with Parkinson's disease and their carers. *Parkinsonism Relat Disord* 2006; **12**(8): 478–85.

80. Wolfrath SC, Borenstein AR, Schwartz S, et al. Use of nutritional supplements in Parkinson's disease patients. *Mov Disord* 2006; **21**(8): 1098–101.

81. Aziz NA, van der Marck MA, Pijl H, et al. Weight loss in neurodegenerative disorders. *J Neurol* 2008; **255**(12): 1872–80.

82. Barichella M, Marczewska A, De NR, et al. Special low-protein foods ameliorate postprandial off in patients with advanced Parkinson's disease. *Mov Disord* 2006; **21**(10): 1682–7.

83. Bronner G, Royter V, Korczyn AD, et al. Sexual dysfunction in Parkinson's disease. *J Sex Marital Ther* 2004; **30**(2): 95–105.

84. Nijkrake MJ, Keus SH, Oostendorp RA, et al. Allied health care in Parkinson's disease: referral, consultation, and professional expertise. *Mov Disord* 2009; **24**(2): 282–6.

85. Munneke M, Keus S, Nijkrake M, et al. Efficiency of evidence-based physiotherapy for Parkinson's disease: the ParkinsonNet trail. *Mov Disord* 2008; **23**(Suppl 1): S220.

Index

abulia 91
acetylcholinesterase inhibitors
19, 69, 91
acquired hepatocerebral
degeneration 104
activities of daily living 143,
146, 148–9
AD (Alzheimer's disease)
15–16, 18, 60
adverse effects
botulinum toxin 45
dopamine agonists 45
levodopa 45
age at presentation
CBD 87
DLB 11, 13
MSA 28
PDCG 108
PSP 65
WD 102
akinesia 129–30
PAGF 62
alcohol use 43
alien limb phenomena (ALP)
81–2, 131
allied health care 142–6
dietary advice 152, 154
multidisciplinary approach
155–6
occupational therapy 45, 47,
69, 146, 153–4
physiotherapy 47, 91, 146–9
sex counseling 154
shortcomings in current
practice 155
social workers 154
speech therapy 47, 91, 146,
149–52
alpha-1-antichymotrypsin
(ACT) 43
Alzheimer's disease (AD)
15–16, 18, 60
amantadine 45, 69, 90
amyloid β 15
amyotrophic lateral sclerosis
(ALS) 78
similar diseases occurring in
the Pacific basin 108–10
anal sphincter EMG 34, 68
animal models 101
MSA 43–4
tauopathies 79

antecollis 33, 148, 152
anticholinergic drugs 45–6, 152
anticonvulsant drugs 90
antidepressants
in CBS/CBD 91
in DLB/PDD 20
in MSA 45
antipsychotic drugs
as cause of parkinsonism
99, 132
in CBS 91
in DLB 13, 20
antisaccade test 68
anxiety 137
aphasia 83, 85, 87
apraxia 11, 81, 91, 131, 137, 154
of speech 85, 133
arginine 35
arm swing 132, 147
aspiration of food 151–2
astrocytes 60, 78
ataxia
ILOCA 34–5, 37
MSA-C 28, 30, 67, 150
spinocerebellar 43, 79, 108
ataxic dysarthria 150
augmentative and alternative
communication (AAC)
151
autoimmune disease 104
autonomic dysfunction 3,
135–6
in DLB 13, 15–16, 20
in MSA 28, 31–4, 38, 40,
135–6
in PD 14, 38, 135
treatment 20, 46–8, 154

baclofen 90
balance see postural instability
ballooned neurons in CBD 76
basal ganglia calcification 108
benzodiazepines 20, 90
Binswanger's disease 107
biomarkers see cerebrospinal
fluid (CSF) markers
bladder dysfunction 135–6,
154
in MSA 28, 33–4, 46–8
treatment 46–8, 154
blepharospasm 69, 132
blinking 61, 68–9, 132

blood pressure see orthostatic
hypotension (OH)
bodig (PDCG) 108–9
botulinum toxin 45, 69, 90,
152
Braak model of ALP pathology
14, 19
bradykinesia 64, 129–30
brainstem atrophy 37, 66, 88
bromocriptine 45

calcification of the basal
ganglia (CBG) 108
calcium channel blockers 100
camptocormia 131
cardiac scintigraphy 15–16,
38, 67
cardiovascular autonomic
dysfunction
see orthostatic
hypotension (OH)
caregivers 13, 143, 146, 154
catheterization, urinary 47
CBD see corticobasal
degeneration
CBG (calcification of the basal
ganglia) 108
CBS see corticobasal syndrome
cerebellar ataxia
ILOCA 34–5, 37
MSA-C 28, 30, 37–8, 67,
150
cerebellar peduncles 37, 66
cerebrospinal fluid (CSF)
markers
CBD 69, 87
DLB 15
MSA 34
PSP 68–9
cerebrovascular disease
see vascular
parkinsonism
cholinesterase inhibitors 19,
69, 91
cinnarizine 100
cirrhosis 102–4
see also Wilson's disease
classification, historical 2–3,
10–11, 27, 75
clinical presentation 1
acquired hepatocerebral
degeneration 104